FAST FACTS FOR THE
CRITICAL CARE NURSE

Critical Care Nursing
in a Nutshell

Michele Angell Landrum, ADN, RN, CCRN, received her associate degree in nursing from the University of Mobile in 1998. She has worked as a travel nurse in various facilities throughout the United States, such as Scripps Memorial Hospital, La Jolla in San Diego and Cedars-Sinai Hospital in Los Angeles. Her specialties include the cardiac care unit, cardiovascular intensive care unit, surgical intensive care unit, emergency room, cardiac catheterization lab, and electrophysiology lab.

Mrs. Landrum is currently employed by Springhill Medical Center in Mobile, Alabama, as a clinical nurse educator with the staff development department.

FAST FACTS FOR THE CRITICAL CARE NURSE

Critical Care Nursing in a Nutshell

Michele Angell Landrum, ADN, RN, CCRN

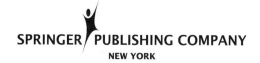

SPRINGER PUBLISHING COMPANY
NEW YORK

Copyright © 2012 Springer Publishing Company, LLC

Springer Publishing Company, LLC
11 West 42nd Street
New York, NY 10036
www.springerpub.com

Acquisitions Editor: Margaret Zuccarini
Composition: Newgen Imaging

ISBN: 978-0-8261-0728-1
eISBN: 978-0-8261-0729-X

11 12 13 14 / 5 4 3 2 1

The author and the publisher of this Work have made every effort to use sources believed to be reliable to provide information that is accurate and compatible with the standards generally accepted at the time of publication. Because medical science is continually advancing, our knowledge base continues to expand. Therefore, as new information becomes available, changes in procedures become necessary. We recommend that the reader always consult current research and specific institutional policies before performing any clinical procedure or administering any drug. The author and publisher shall not be liable for any special, consequential, or exemplary damages resulting, in whole or in part, from the readers' use of, or reliance on, the information contained in this book. The publisher has no responsibility for the persistence or accuracy of URLs for external or third-party Internet Web sites referred to in this publication and does not guarantee that any content on such Web sites is, or will remain, accurate or appropriate.

Cataloging-in-Publication Data is on file at the Library of Congress.

Special discounts on bulk quantities of our books are available to corporations, professional associations, pharmaceutical companies, health care organizations, and other qualifying groups. If you are interested in a custom book, including chapters from more than one of our titles, we can provide that service as well.

For details, please contact:
Special Sales Department, Springer Publishing Company, LLC
11 West 42nd Street, 15th Floor, New York, NY 10036-8002
Phone: 877-687-7476 or 212-431-4370; Fax: 212-941-7842
Email: sales@springerpub.com

Printed in the United States of America by Hamilton Printing.

This book is dedicated to my husband Ted for his continued love, support, and encouragement, and also to my sons Carter and Cody, for it is their love, joy, patience, and understanding that makes every day a blessing.

—M.A.L.

Contents

Preface

Critical care nursing is one of the most challenging nursing options available. It requires astute assessment skills, extremely specialized training, the ability to multitask, adaptability, top-notch communication skills, attention to detail while seeing the big picture, positive coping techniques, and numerous other traits. This guide is intended to help make practicing as a critical care nurse a little easier.

The guide is designed to work as an assistant. It includes guidelines for documentation, advance directives, organ donation, withdrawal of treatment, and palliative care. Basic assessment and procedural skills are detailed, along with more in-depth acute care practices, such as managing an intra-aortic balloon pump. Aseptic technique, isolation precautions, IV therapy, central venous line and pulmonary artery catheter care, and continuous renal replacement therapy are explained in an easy-to-read manner. Applications pertaining to individual ICUs are also included.

Several of the topics in this guide apply to current nursing concerns nationwide. Joint Commission topics such as proper patient identification are discussed. Isolation precautions and personal protective equipment applications recommended by the Centers for Disease Control and Prevention are detailed, and information about performing palliative care in the ICU is provided.

This guide can work as both a training manual and a reference tool. Keep it at the bedside for a quick refresher on ICU nursing implementations and to help troubleshoot mechanical devices used in the critical care unit.

Please keep in mind that while this book was compiled using numerous resources, it does not contain every possible ICU intervention or procedural guideline. Refer to facility protocol and manufacturer recommendations, along with physicians' orders, as needed. Personal and patient safety is always of primary concern.

Michele Angell Landrum, ADN, RN, CCRN

Acknowledgments

Thank you to all the wonderful nurses whom I have had the pleasure to work among. It is through education, preceptorship, training, and teamwork that I was able to experience amazing medical treatments and nursing practice. I happily share the knowledge gained as a travel nurse, working with some of the best nurses, physicians, and support staff in the country.

Much appreciation goes to Stephanie and Ben Kunz, Diane Pike, Anjanetta Davis, MSN, RN, CNL, Scott Wilson, RN, and Beth Beck, MT (ASCP), CIC for their support and encouragement during the writing of this guide, and to Bimbola F. Akintade PhD©, ACNP, CCRN, for a careful review of the content.

Finally, special thanks to my family. Ted, Carter, Cody, and Vera (Mom), you have been incredibly patient, supportive, and understanding during this busy time. Each of you mean more to me than you will ever know. Thank you.

FAST FACTS FOR THE CRITICAL CARE NURSE

Critical Care Nursing in a Nutshell

Foundations of Critical Care

Critical Care Nursing Overview

INTRODUCTION

The American Association of Critical Care Nurses (AACN) defines critical care nursing as "a specialty within nursing that deals specifically with human responses to life-threatening problems" (April 2010). Critical care units range from open-heart recovery units, burn units, and neurologic intensive care units (ICUs) to surgical ICUs, medical ICUs, and cardiac care units. All have distinct qualities while sharing several similar attributes.

Nurses who thrive in these areas are highly specialized and well trained, assess patients efficiently, and provide appropriate, proficient, culturally relevant, and emotionally sensitive care for both the patient and his or her family. These are the core values of critical care nursing.

Critical care nurses maintain the highest quality of care for patients, interact diplomatically within the medical system, and take care of themselves and their families.

In this chapter, you will learn:

1. The qualifications for critical care nurses and available certifications.
2. The different types of critical care units and their patient care sets and equipment.
3. Self-care guidelines for nurses working in a critical care environment.

QUALIFICATIONS

Most nurses who are interested in a critical care position already possess the appropriate requirements. These include

1. An active registered nursing license in the state of employment.
2. An unencumbered nursing license in the state of employment.
   a. A license not currently subject to discipline by any board of nursing.
   b. A license without provisions and/or conditions for nursing practice.

While the actual requirements for critical care nursing are few, the qualities desired by hospitals are numerous. Interviews with several directors and managers of various critical care units regarding the type of nurses they hire revealed several key characteristics. Being organized and able to keep up in a fast-paced environment were frequently mentioned, with quite a few managers adding that "being able to think on one's feet" is a valuable trait. A great resume and a history of providing ethical and competent patient care were stressed. One director mentioned that **strong clinical skills and references are important for all applicants,** and that for new graduates without much work history, a productive practicum or clinical experience, with references, is a must.

Critical care nurses share many traits with others practicing throughout the nursing spectrum. They are organized, ethical, proficient, caring, humane, respectful, eager to learn, cool under pressure, and confident. **Nurses always keep what is best for the patient foremost, thereby ensuring that proper care is given.** Once hired, a critical care nurse has hospital and unit orientations. During the unit orientation, a nurse is assigned a preceptor, who begins teaching critical care techniques. **Education and training must be ongoing** throughout critical care nursing to ensure up-to-date skills and competency.

CERTIFICATIONS

Nurses working in the critical care field can obtain several certifications. Most of these are offered by the AACN. Certified Critical Care Registered Nurse (CCRN) accreditation is the most common; however, only about 50,000 nurses hold this title nationwide (AACN, March 2010). This certification is further specialized into adult, pediatric, and neonatal care, or any combination of the three.

Applicants for the CCRN exam must meet eligibility requirements prior to testing. The test is based on practice analysis in critical care, and achieving certification is a prestigious accomplishment. Once a nurse has passed the exam, CCRN is maintained via a renewal policy every 3 years, if all requirements are met.

Additional subspecialty certifications exist for nurses who have CCRN certification. **Cardiac medicine certification (CMC) and cardiac surgery certification (CSC) are available to nurses who meet the requirements corresponding to the subspecialty. Both require the passing of a certification exam.**

TYPES OF CRITICAL CARE UNITS

All critical care units, commonly referred to as ICUs, have similarities; however, several items and situations vary according to the particular type of critical care area. The number of patient beds or rooms is generally the biggest variant. A unit may have 2 beds or 25 to 30 beds, depending on the hospital size, location, and specialty demand.

=========================*FAST FACTS in a NUTSHELL*

Common Characteristics of Critical Care Units

1. A nurse-to-patient ratio of 1:1 or 1:2.
2. Critically ill patients.
3. Patients with multiple diagnoses.
4. Specialized equipment: Continuous EKG, blood pressure, and oxygen saturation monitors; multiple IV pumps, arterial lines, pulmonary artery catheter, endotracheal tubes, ventilators, chest tubes, urinary catheters, central venous lines, and nasogastric tubes and/or g-tubes.
5. Isolation precautions.
6. Restricted visiting hours.
7. Bedside computers for documentation.

The type of patients in intensive care varies according to the facility, unit type, and staff and bed availability. Usually, a facility has a general ICU that is a catch-all for most types of patients and a surgical ICU for post-surgical patients. Both utilize most of the equipment mentioned, as well as other items, such as an intra-aortic balloon pump (IABP) and a continuous venovenous hemodialysis (CVVHD) machine. Various other types of critical care units also exist.

- The **surgical intensive care unit (SICU) is where patients recover after extremely invasive surgery,** such as a Whipple procedure, orthopedic reconstruction, or complex abdominal repair. They often have additional medical conditions that require close monitoring and special treatment.
- The neurologic intensive care unit (NICU), is another area with highly specialized care and equipment.

Patients in the NICU require detailed care that pertains to their neurological status. They might have experienced a stroke, exhibit increased intracranial pressure (ICP), have suffered acute head trauma, or be comatose. An ICP monitor and/or drain is often inserted and maintained in this patient care setting.

- The cardiac care unit (CCU) is common in most hospitals and is for patients experiencing some type of cardiac issue. They might be pre- or post-heart catheterization, suffering from chest pain, have experienced an acute myocardial infarction, or even be pre- or post-open-heart surgery. An IABP often is used in the CCU. CCRNs with a CMC subspecialty certification might work in the CCU.

- The cardiovascular intensive care unit (CVICU) is generally for post-cardiac bypass patients. However, other patients may be admitted to this unit, including those with post-op thoracic aneurysm repair, abdominal aneurysm repair, and thoracotomies. IABPs, left ventricular assist devices (LVADs), biventricular assist devices (BIVADs), and CVVHD devices are often used in this unit. CVICU nurses may have CCRN certification with a CSC subspecialty certification.

- The transplant unit, where post-organ-transplant patients recover, trains its nurses specifically for this patient population. There are extremely rigid parameters that must be maintained for such patients, as well as infection control protocols. Multiple types of equipment and monitoring systems are in this unit.

- The burn unit is for multiple types of burn victims. Patients suffering from thermal, scalding, chemical, or electrical burns need specific treatment.

- The trauma ICU is for patients with various types of injuries and several diagnoses. The equipment in this unit can range from a simple arterial line to CVVHD to orthopedic traction. Nurses in the trauma ICU must be prepared for any and all types of wounds and patient care.

The critical care units mentioned above are explored in the following chapters, which explain the specific guidelines, equipment, and skills utilized.

While each specialty unit tries to use open beds for patients meeting its specialty, **ICU nurses must be prepared to care for any type of critically ill or injured patient who may require an ICU bed.** A facility may engage any available room when the critical care areas are close to capacity.

SELF-CARE FOR THE CRITICAL CARE NURSE

Working in the field of nursing is difficult and demanding, but nevertheless very rewarding. Critical care nursing has adrenaline highs and corresponding lows often surpassing those of other nursing practice areas. Critical care nurses must learn how to handle and relieve stress to perform their job effectively.

═══════════════════════════*FAST FACTS in a NUTSHELL*

Strategies to Relieve Stress

1. Stay hydrated and eat well-balanced meals.
2. Exercise and maintain flexibility.
3. Get 7–8 hours of sleep daily.
4. Separate work and home life; spend off-duty time with family and friends.
5. Maintain a positive outlook.
6. Participate in hobbies outside of work.
7. Maintain a sense of humor.
8. Take 3 seconds to just breathe.
9. Discuss concerns about patients, coworkers, and/or doctors with the nurse manger.
10. Seek counseling, if needed, to handle grief, emotions, and stress.

In addition to following a healthful diet and managing stress while remaining physically and emotionally fit, ICU nurses should see their own physicians at least once a year, stay up-to-date on immunizations, and receive annual flu shots.

By actively providing self-care, nurses improve the quality of care that they provide to their patients and loved ones. All the strategies mentioned will help keep stress at a minimum; however, there is one key to performing well and making the best decisions while on the job: **Do what is best for the patient.** By honoring this mantra, nurses will ask questions when needed, seek appropriate consultation, and provide the right type of care, all while exhibiting great nursing skills and protecting their licenses.

2

The Importance of Documentation

INTRODUCTION

Accurate and timely documentation of care is required in all areas of nursing. It is a legal driving force in every nursing discipline and patient care environment. Documentation is the method used to describe, monitor, manage, and modify patient care. The format used is varied and acronyms abound. Each facility sets its own guidelines for how documentation is performed. In today's technological society, computers and electronic medical records (EMRs) are commonly utilized.

Clear, concise documentation is essential. The nursing process is the foundation for patient care and documentation.

In this chapter, you will review the following:

1. The five steps in the nursing process.
2. The basic rules of documenting patient care.
3. The definition of *malpractice* and documentation strategies that can help to prevent its occurrence.

NURSING STANDARDS OF PRACTICE

Nursing is based on standards that define, guide, and evaluate nursing practice along with its suggested outcomes. The American Nurses Association (ANA) describes **six core standards of practice**, including

1. *Assessment:* Collection of data.
2. *Diagnosis:* Analysis of data to determine nursing diagnosis.
3. *Outcome Identification:* Identification of expected outcomes specific to the patient and/or situation.
4. *Planning:* Development of a plan detailing interventions aimed to achieve expected outcomes.
5. *Implementation:* Performance of the interventions noted in the plan of care.
6. *Evaluation:* Evaluation of the patient's progress toward achievement of expected outcomes (American Nurses Association. (2004). *Nursing: Scope and standards of practice.* Washington, DC: Author).

THE NURSING PROCESS

The ANA describes the nursing process as **the "essential core of practice for the registered nurse"** (April 2010). The five steps of the nursing process are as follows:

1. *Assessment:* The gathering of psychosocial, physical, spiritual, economic, and lifestyle factors by:
   a. Interviewing the patient and/or family members.
   b. Reviewing past medical history and records.
   c. Completing a physical examination and reviewing current patient data.
2. *Diagnosis:* The issue on which the nursing care plan is based. The nursing diagnosis is the clinical judgment regarding the patient's response to actual or possible medical problems. It is based on the assessment.

3. *Planning and Outcomes:* Are detailed in the nursing care plan by:
   a. Assigning priorities, if the patient has multiple nursing diagnoses.
   b. Setting short- and long-term goals that are patient-oriented and measurable.
   c. Including assessment and diagnosis details.
   d. Stating appropriate nursing interventions and corresponding medical orders.
   e. Utilizing a standardized or computerized care plan or clinical pathway as a guideline, if appropriate.
4. *Implementation:* The performance of nursing care according to the care plan by
   a. Documenting the care provided to the patient properly.
   b. Performing treatment in a way that minimizes complications and life-threatening issues.
   c. Involving patients, families, caregivers, and other members of the health care team as their abilities and patient safety allow.
5. *Evaluation:* The process of evaluating the status of the patient and the effectiveness of the treatment. The plan of care may be modified if warranted.

The five steps of the nursing process drive how a nurse determines, completes, and documents patient care, education, health care team interaction, and just about every activity performed in the workplace.

The AACN Standards of Care and AACN Scope of Practice further define the critical care nurse's role in quality nursing practice, expected professionalism, education, collegiality, ethical situations, collaboration with the patient, family, and health care team, clinical inquiries, utilizing appropriate resources, and leadership (Bell, 2008). Additional information is provided on the AACN Web site (www.AACN.org) and in "*AACN Scope and Standards for Acute and Critical Care Nursing Practice.*"

DOCUMENTATION

Critical care documentation requires a basic understanding of the nursing process and how to utilize a care plan. All nurses learn how to complete focus notes, DARP notes, SOAP notes, or some variation of these types of documentation as student nurses. However, most **hospitals, including their critical care units, now use computerized documentation.** By 2014, the federal government will require all health care providers to use EMRs (Cover, July 2010). The change from paper to computer-based documentation is an important advantage in critical care nursing.

Numerous software companies sell EMR programs that incorporate almost all activities that nurses and other members of the health care team perform. This generally makes documentation much easier, more standardized, and more accurate. A nurse can easily access a patient's chart, according to the particular program guidelines, locate the page for the assessment, dressing change, patient education, or other procedure that he or she has completed, and check boxes containing the correct information. A blank box is offered where additional documentation can be entered, such as details and other items pertaining to tasks performed. A similar situation exists for documenting medications given using an Electronic Medication Administration Record (EMAR).

EMRs and EMARs are designed to make documentation easier, as they have programs and pages for numerous situations that occur in critical care units. However, documenting all the required assessments, care plans, EMARs, physician orders, and multiple other components can be a daunting task. A nurse must **remember the nursing process, liability, safety, and patient care when documenting.** It is always necessary to "save," or store, the information after inputting it properly.

Each hospital should have a tech team available 24/7 whose responsibility is to help staff resolve documentation problems involving EMRs and EMARs.

═══════════════════════════════*FAST FACTS in a NUTSHELL*

A critical care nurse must be aware that despite all the technology employed in the ICU, the rule, **"If it was not documented, it was not done"** still holds true. EMRs and EMARs are the center of communication among nursing staff, medical staff, therapists, the lab, the pharmacy, and all other members of the health care team. If something is not documented, it cannot be verified and evaluated properly.

If an item, procedure, complication, patient/family situation, or other activity is not on the EMR, find an appropriate place to add the issue in a free-text location. Make references to it when documenting in other areas. Case Study 2.1 illustrates a documentation situation that occurs commonly.

Case Study 2.1

A patient accidentally removed a peripheral, hep-locked IV from her right hand while trying to use the TV remote control. Quickly, the nurse assigned to the patient assessed the situation. Recognizing the potential risk for infection and bleeding as nursing diagnoses, she methodically developed a plan of care according to facility guidelines.

Implementing the plan, the RN donned gloves and properly applied pressure to the site until hemostasis. She then placed a small sterile bandage over the site. Evaluating the area, she noted no hematoma.

Given that the site was the only IV access and the physician orders required an IV while the patient remained hospitalized, the nurse inserted a #20 peripheral IV into the patient's left forearm on the initial

Continued

Continued

stick, after using hospital protocol for site preparation. The IV was secured with a tegaderm and was patent, exhibiting positive blood return. The IV was flushed with 10 cc normal saline, per policy, and heplocked per physician order. The patient had no known allergies. The IV was secured with one piece of plastic tape.

Patient education was completed regarding the need for the IV, as well as, how the patient might avoid inadvertently removing it. The patient tolerated the procedure well, acknowledging understanding of the procedure, IV education, and care.

After completing and evaluating the procedure, the nurse accessed the patient's EMR to document the changes, implementations, and outcome. Several of the actions performed were readily available to check off, but there was no area discussing the appearance of the initial site after the IV was removed. A free-text box was an option on the bottom of the IV screen. The nurse added details about the appearance of the site and how the IV was removed to ensure adequate documentation. Finally, she accessed the patient's EMAR, located the page that pertained to peripheral IVs, and noted the site change.

This example demonstrates proper nursing process and documentation, patient safety concerns, and good communication. With the documentation of what transpired in two places, other nurses who care for the patient will note the IV site change and be able to refer to the other page where IV information is found, to read the details of the situation.

MALPRACTICE

Critical care nurses must document all aspects of patient care according to the nursing process while following each step of the process in their daily practice. Patient and family education must also be documented. Restraints, whether physical or chemical, require strict documentation following facility specific guidelines. **The best way to ensure proper patient care and outcomes, while avoiding malpractice issues, is to maintain detailed-oriented, appropriate documentation and provide proficient care that is focused on patient safety and within the scope of critical care nursing practice.**

═══════════════════════════════════*FAST FACTS in a NUTSHELL*

Webster's Dictionary defines *malpractice* as a "dereliction of professional duty or a failure to exercise an ordinary degree of professional skill...or rendering professional services which results in injury, loss, or damage. *Negligence* is defined as "failure to exercise the care that a reasonably prudent person would exercise in like circumstances" (July 2010).

To avoid negligence, as well as, malpractice issues, nurses must practice according to the Nurse Practice Act (NPA) of the state in which care is provided. Guidelines can generally be found via the state's Board of Nursing or Board of Health. It is important that nurses be familiar with state laws regarding nurses' legal rights, responsibilities, and scope of practice, as well as violations, disciplinary actions, and penalties. Knowledge of these guidelines allows nurses to care for patients to the best of their abilities while providing competent care.

It is up to each individual nurse to decide if he or she wants to buy a malpractice insurance policy. Investigation and research of the numerous companies that offer such polices is suggested to determine which company and policy suits the practitioner.

A nurse should be aware of his or her skill, experience, and expertise level, seeking appropriate collaboration, education, training, and/or assistance when necessary. Following the chain of command when problems arise is important. **Asking questions while providing optimal care, education, and outcomes for patients and their family members is key to nursing practice.** Maintaining one's own safety when implementing patient and family care is also paramount.

3

Advance Directives and Organ Donation

INTRODUCTION

A critical care unit is an exciting, adventurous place to work. Unfortunately, there are some drawbacks that arise when caring for critically ill patients and their families. The most emotionally and physically challenging aspect of nursing, a patient's death, is often encountered in an ICU. While end-of-life care is a challenge for hospital staff and frightening for the patient and family, numerous things can be done to help the patient, family, and staff cope positively with an impending death.

In this chapter you will learn:

1. The definition of a living will versus a medical durable power of attorney.
2. Eye and organ donation guidelines.
3. Guidelines related to nursing interventions for the care of donor patients.

ADVANCE DIRECTIVES

The Federal Patient Self-Determination Act (PSDA) of 1990 requires each state to develop a law for advance directives. It also requires all health care facilities to:

1. Provide written information describing the directives.
2. Distribute written information detailing patient's rights to make health care decisions that include:
   a. The right to accept or refuse medical treatment.
   b. The right to accept or refuse surgical treatment.
   c. The right to develop an advance directive.
3. Provide a copy of their policies for the implementation of patients' rights.
4. Document whether patients have advance directives in their medical records.
5. Not "condition care" or discriminate against patients based on advance directives.
6. Comply with the state law regarding advance directives.
7. Provide education to their staff and local area explaining advance directives.

With these laws and mandates in place, it is important for critical care nurses to clearly understand how advance directives work. **There are two types of advance directives, though they may be combined. In a living will, a person details what type of medical treatment he or she would or would not want if he or she were to become incompetent.** A living will may be general or extremely specific, detailing certain interventions such as mechanical ventilation, artificial nutrition, or cardio-pulmonary resuscitation (CPR). A living will does not indicate a health care representative.

A medical durable power of attorney, or health care power of attorney, documents the person whom a person names as his or her health care agent, or proxy. This person should be 18 years of age or older and, ideally, guided by a living will. The health care proxy has the same rights regarding health care decisions that a patient has prior to becoming incompetent. However, the laws differ in some states regarding do-not-resuscitate (DNR) orders and medical durable power of attorney decisions.

═══════════════════════════════════════*FAST FACTS in a NUTSHELL*

Both a living will and medical durable power of attorney are written documents completed by a person while he or she is competent. Most states do not require a specific form for an advance directive or that the form be notarized; however, it should be witnessed by two adults and signed by the person. If the person is unable to sign, someone else may do so other than the witnesses or a health care provider. Nurses should become familiar with the state laws and facility policies where they practice.

Most states, facilities, and physicians recommend that people complete advance directives long before they are ever needed. These documents help health care providers fulfill the wishes of their patients and bring peace of mind to patients and families.

EYE AND ORGAN DONATION

Eye and organ donation are extremely important. According to the United Network for Organ Sharing (UNOS), on July 16, 2010, there were 107,952 people in the United States awaiting an organ transplant (2010). **The waiting list grows longer each day, while the number of potential donors does not.** The reasons for the low number of donors are numerous, and many myths and misconceptions abound. Examples of myths and misconceptions, which medical professionals know are unfounded, include the following:

1. If a physician knows that a patient is an organ donor, he or she will not work as hard to save the patient.

2. Being rich and famous improves a patient's place on the transplant list.
3. Listing "organ donor" on a driver's license or having a donor card is all that is needed to be a donor.
4. The only organs that can be transplanted are the heart, liver, and/or kidneys.
5. Most patients with a medical history are not fit to donate organs.
6. Older patients are not eligible to donate organs.
7. The family of the donor is charged a fee if organs are donated.
8. If the organs of a patient are donated, the body is changed in such a way that it is unsuitable for viewing at the funeral.
9. Most religions do not allow organ donation.

(Adapted from UNOS, 2004, "Common Myths of Organ Donation.")

========================*FAST FACTS in a NUTSHELL*

While a patient may not be suitable for heart donation, other organs often can be used, such as the corneas, lungs, liver, pancreas, kidneys, skin, bone, bone marrow, cartilage, tendons, fascia, and/or dura mater.

It is the responsibility of the hospital staff, local and state organ bank representatives, and UNOS to educate patients, family members, and the public. In 2004, the Joint Commission on Accreditation of Health care Organizations published the book *Health Care at the Crossroads: Strategies for Narrowing the Organ Donation Gap and Protecting Patients*. This book contains information about organ donation, suggested improvements for hospitals, and follow-up guidelines regarding donation.

Critical care nurses often encounter situations where eye and/or organ donation is a possibility. **It is important to provide emotional support and education to the family while attempting to honor the patient's wishes, either for or against donation.** According to the 2006 Universal

Anatomical Gift Act (UAGA), organs of a patient who indicated prior to death that he or she wished to participate in organ donation, such as on a driver's license, must be considered for donation. The UAGA also specifies that if a patient previously signed a refusal for eye and/or organ donation, family members or the health care proxy cannot override the patient's wishes and should not be requested to do so (Foreman et al., 2010).

Once it is clear that a patient requested to be a donor or if there is no indication of the patient's wishes in this regard, **medical suitability for eye and/or organ donation must be considered before approaching the family** to prevent undue emotional distress.

=== *FAST FACTS in a NUTSHELL*

Some people request that their body be donated to "science" for medical research. Most research centers accept bodies and organs regardless of illness, pathology, or cause of death. A person usually has contact information for the facility that will be accepting his or her body detailed in an advance directive.

Most hospitals have policies outlining their organ donation/procurement process. Some general guidelines are as follows:

1. A potential organ donor is identified.
2. An organ procurement organization (OPO), such as a state organ center or eye bank, is notified that a death is imminent. Discuss the patient's status with family members in an open, unbiased manner to allow them time to make informed decisions regarding eye and organ donation, and to express emotions about the patient's imminent death. Answer all questions honestly. Seek help from the OPO, if needed.
3. When the OPO is contacted, the medical team caring for the patient is asked various questions, including the

patient's age, current status, and medical history, to determine preliminary suitability for donation.

4. A physician who meets the health care institution's guidelines for the appropriate skill set, training, and expertise regarding neurological status must make a declaration of brain death, defined as irreversible loss of all brain function, based on both clinical and radiological evidence. A second opinion may be required.

5. Written consent is completed and witnessed once the family has had time to process the situation with support and education from the OPO representative, hospital staff, and/or clergy. A release from the medical examiner may also be required. Once this paperwork is complete, the patient is officially a "donor."

6. The donor's true medical suitability must be determined through a detailed medical and social history, a complete organ systems review, and lab work. OPOs and eye, organ, and tissue banks help this process flow smoothly.

7. Donor management care must be provided throughout the evaluation period. Medications, respiratory care, and IV fluids are given to the donor to maximize the integrity of the organs and tissues for procurement.

8. The organ procurement procedure is performed using sterile technique once medical suitability is determined. The organs are preserved with a solution, then transferred into sterile bags and stored on ice in coolers. Specially trained transplant teams are used to transport the organs according to the OPO directions. Tissue recovery takes place similarly after the viable organs have been procured.

9. Disposition of the donor's body, per facility guidelines and the wishes of the patient and/or family, occurs.

10. Prompt follow-up occurs, with OPOs sending a letter to the donor's family detailing information about the recipients of their loved one's organs. Information regarding the organ recipients and the amazing outcome of the

hard work completed by the team is provided to the facility and staff where the organs were harvested. The recipients' identities are not revealed.

(Adapted from U.S. Department of Veterans Affairs, Veterans Health Administration, 2009; University of Miami, Leonard M. Miller School of Medicine, Department of Surgery, Life Alliance Organ Recovery Agency. *The organ donation process*, 2010; Wingate & Wiegand, 2008.)

Grief counseling is often available to donor families. Some OPOs have ceremonies throughout the year to honor the extraordinary gift of life that the donor and family provided.

4

Withdrawal of Treatment and Palliative Care

INTRODUCTION

Emotional support is a key component of end-of-life care and is important for the patient, family, caregivers, and ICU staff. Certain strategies and guidelines can help ease the stress and emotional turmoil associated with imminent death and end-of-life care. Guidelines for withdrawal of treatment, palliative care, and the generalized protocol for a terminal wean can help facilitate a "good" death.

In this chapter you will learn:

1. Guidelines for the withdrawal of medical treatment.
2. The general protocol for a *terminal wean*.
3. How to provide palliative care.
4. How to emotionally support patients and family when death is imminent.
5. Self-care guidelines for nurses providing end-of-life care.

WITHDRAWAL OF MEDICAL TREATMENT

Once the hospital physicians and the patient's family and/or health care proxy decide that additional medical intervention would be futile, **medical treatment can be withdrawn.** This includes ventilation support, nutrition, IV fluids, antibiotics, and/or blood products. **Withdrawal of medical treatment is an emotional subject for both the family and the staff.**

Prior to withdrawal of treatment, the physicians, nurses, clergy, social workers, and other hospital support staff should provide clear details to family members regarding the process and allow them time to absorb this information. Some clinicians suggest using the term "choosing comfort" because families tend to find it easier to understand and less emotionally taxing than some other terms (Foreman et al., 2010).

═══════════════════════════════*FAST FACTS in a NUTSHELL*

To help the family cope with the situation, it is important to assure them that

1. The cause of death is the underlying disease, not the withdrawal of treatment.
2. Medication will be administered to maintain the patient's comfort and prevent suffering.
3. Staff will continue to care for the patient. He or she will not be neglected.

TERMINAL WEAN

The withdrawal of ventilator support from an incurably ill patient is often referred to as a terminal wean. For the family, the nurse usually follows these guidelines:

1. Rely on a properly trained nurse and respiratory therapist who perform this procedure at the patient's bedside.

2. Determine whether family members wish to remain with the patient during the terminal wean process and spend time with the patient after death. These questions should be asked in a caring, understanding, and nonjudgmental way.
3. Ensure that the room is as comfortable as possible. Provide chairs, tissues, and as much privacy as possible. Be readily available to address family needs and/or provide measures and medications for the patient's comfort.
4. Facilitate any family requests for spiritual/clergy support.
5. Prepare the family for what to expect during the terminal wean process in a clear, concise, caring manner. Symptoms that families can expect the patient to exhibit are decreasing consciousness, restlessness, reflexive movements, changes in breathing patterns, audible secretions, and cool and discolored extremities.
6. Encourage family members to touch and speak to the patient and express any feelings they are experiencing. After the patient expires, allow the family to spend time in the room.

(Adapted from Foreman, Milisen, & Fulmer, 2010; Wingate & Wiegand, 2008; Wyckoff, Houghton, & LePage, 2009.)

The facility and its practitioners follow a specific protocol, which usually includes:

1. Document conversations with the family and other health care team members.
2. Consider organ donation prior to treatment withdrawal.
3. Maintain IV access site for palliative care medication administration.
4. Remove monitoring equipment that is not needed for patient comfort.
5. Hold all neuromuscular blocking medications, providing adequate reversal time.
6. Administer pain/anxiety medications 30 minutes prior to initiation of ventilator withdrawal.

7. Remove restraints.
8. Decide between gradual or immediate ventilator withdrawal:
   a. Gradual ventilator withdrawal: Reduction of the respiratory rate (RR) of the ventilator by 2–3 breaths per minute, at 15 minute intervals, until the RR of the vent is zero. Next, reduce positive-end-expiratory pressure (PEEP) and pressure support (PS) until the patient exhibits spontaneous respiration.
   b. Immediate ventilator withdrawal: The ventilator is withdrawn without changes in RR, PEEP, or PS.
9. Position patient upright, when possible.
10. Administer antisecretory medication, such as hycoscyamine (Anaspaz), if ordered.
11. Administer haloperidol (Haldol) or midazolam (Versed) for terminal restlessness, if ordered.
12. Begin ventilator withdrawal.
13. Continuously monitor the patient for signs and symptoms of pain, respiratory distress, agitation, or anxiety.
14. Administer medications for pain, respiratory distress, agitation, and/or anxiety, as needed, to keep patient comfortable.
15. Extubate the patient, if ordered.
16. Notify the physician when spontaneous respirations have ceased.

(Adapted from Foreman et al., 2010; Saint Thomas Hospital, 2000; Stillwell, 2006; Wingate & Wiegand, 2008.)

FAST FACTS in a NUTSHELL

Withdrawal of ventilator support for a patient is rarely a medical examiner's case. If it is, follow hospital protocol for removal of lines, chest and endotracheal tubes, and any other applicable modality before, during, and after medical treatment withdrawal.

PALLIATIVE CARE

Once the health care team and family determine that continued medical intervention and treatment would be futile, the transition to palliative care begins. **Palliative care is the active total care of patients with an advanced illness** (*Lippincott Manual of Nursing Practice,* 9th ed.). During this phase of critical care, the focus shifts to the patient's quality of life and comfort level. **A team of physicians, nurses, social workers, and spiritual advisors work to make the patient and family as comfortable as possible.**

If the patient is able, discuss requests and preferences. Are specific family members to visit? Does the patient want any religious and/or cultural practices to be observed? **Encourage the patient to express any emotions that he or she is experiencing.** Listen in an open manner. Answer questions honestly.

Frequently, once care turns to palliation in the ICU, the patient's health status has progressed to such a serious point that the patient is no longer able to make decisions for him- or herself. **The family then becomes the focus of the health care team's emotional support.** It is important to provide education regarding care, symptoms, and medical management. Assure the family that medications will be provided to alleviate pain and anxiety, and that the patient will not be neglected because of the choice to withhold or withdraw medical treatment. A comfortable environment encourages family members to interact with and care for the patient. Allow them to express all emotions.

In the critical care unit, managing the symptoms that patients encounter during end-of-life care is paramount. **Pain, dyspnea, restlessness, and/or terminal delirium are the major symptoms that occur. Skin care is also a priority with these patients.**

Pain is treated with a combination of medications. Nonsteroidal anti-inflammatory drugs (NSAIDS), opioids (primarily morphine), and corticosteroids are used to treat pain during palliative care. Antidepressants are also often given to relieve neuropathic pain. It is important to try to identify and eradicate sources of pain. Undertreatment of pain is often reported by family members; however, this is not an acceptable outcome. Vigilance regarding pain control is required when providing palliative care.

Position the patient for comfort and reassess frequently for pain. Because the patient is often unable to express pain on a 1–10 scale, observe facial expressions, respirations, moaning or groaning, and consolability (American Medical Directors Association, 2004). During end-of-life care, dosages of certain medications, such as morphine, may exceed those in general critical care nursing practice.

Dyspnea occurs in almost all patients undergoing end-of-life care. This is uncomfortable for the patient to experience and for the family to observe. Diuretics and morphine lessen congestion, while anxiolytics help to reduce anxiety. A trial of low-dose oxygen may reduce dyspnea; however, it is not used to improve O_2 saturation levels. The patient should be positioned upright in bed, if possible, to maximize lung capacity. One inch of nitroglycerin paste applied to the chest wall may improve orthopnea. Hycoscyamine sulfate can be given in an attempt to reduce audible secretions. If wheezing is noted, bronchodilators are often administered.

Proper skin care and hygiene are essential during end-of-life care, as they maximize comfort and assure both patient and family that care is ongoing. ICU skin care protocols should be followed. Bathe the patient daily and as needed. Use facility or wound-care team moisturizers, as suggested. Turn the patient every 2 hours, or as needed, based on pain and/or discomfort. Use a low-pressure mattress system, if available and if patient condition dictates need. Provide frequent oral care.

Patients undergoing end-of-life care often exhibit terminal delirium and restlessness. Other signs and symptoms include nonpurposeful motor activity, changing level of consciousness, cognitive failure, agitation, and hallucinations. Haloperidol (Haldol), olanzapine (Zyprexa), risperidone (Risperdal), midazolam (Versed), and/or chlorpromazine

(Thorazine) may be administered, if ordered, to combat these symptoms and provide comfort to the patient.

===========================*FAST FACTS in a NUTSHELL*

A patient close to death may experience nearing-death awareness (NDA). Deceased loved ones may appear to the patient and "speak." Other visions might also occur. NDA is different from terminal delirium, primarily because the patient is not distressed or afraid of the visions. Their message is usually symbolic and might also be directed to family members. Explain to them and the patient that this type of experience is normal (Foreman et al., 2010).

EMOTIONAL SUPPORT OF THE FAMILY

End-of-life care involves many clinical skills and requires positive emotional support for the patient and family. Remember to:

1. Allow family members to spend as much time as possible with the patient prior to and after death.
2. Provide the family access to clergy or other spiritual advisors if they request it. Attempt to honor the religious practices of the patient and family.
3. Be emotionally and physically available to discuss the patient's status, providing full disclosure of the situation.
4. Provide time for family members to ask questions, express emotions, and grieve.
5. Invite the family to participate in the final care following death of their loved one. Some family members will opt in; others will not.
6. Be sensitive to the possibility that a family member might need to actually hear medical personnel state that the patient has expired.
7. Offer follow-up care that might include

a. A meeting of the family and physician or health care team.
b. A simple card or phone call from the health care team.
c. Information about the facility's bereavement program and support groups for those who have experienced the death of a loved one.
d. Contact with a social worker for referral to post-hospital emotional support.

(Adapted from Foreman, Milisen, & Fulmer, 2010; Nettina, 2010; Stillwell, 2006; Wingate & Wiegand, 2008; Wyckoff, Houghton, & LePage, 2009.)

HEALTH CARE TEAM EMOTIONAL SUPPORT

Working in the critical care unit is physically demanding and emotionally taxing. It is a labor of love. Nurses, as well as the rest of the health care team, are concerned about the patients and families they care for and tend to forget about their own needs, especially when dealing with end-of-life issues such as organ donation, withdrawal of medical treatment, and palliative care.

Critical care nurses must remember to take the steps necessary to support their own physical and emotional health. Education regarding end-of-life care protocols and expectations is one way to improve understanding of the dying process. Actually participating in such care produces positive experiences related to patient and family comfort and satisfaction. Some important considerations include:

1. Exercising moderately, eating a well-balanced diet, and staying hydrated to maintain physical health and support the ability to provide excellent care
2. Participating in activities outside of work, enjoying hobbies, and relaxing with friends and family to maintain positive emotional health

3. The support of clergy, social workers, bereavement counselors, and psychosocial support staff to improve coping skills, find emotional release, and manage grief

Additional advice and guidelines regarding palliative care in the ICU can be found at www.capc.org/ipal-icu. The Center to Advance Palliative Care manages the Website with support from the National Institutes of Health/National Institute on Aging.

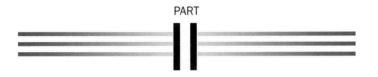

Critical Care Basics

5

Basic Patient Care in the Critical Care Setting

INTRODUCTION

Critical care nursing involves skills, education, and training above and beyond nursing-school basics; however, the steps in the nursing process and patient care are the same. The first step in patient care is assessment, which includes a review of the patient's past medical history, cultural and family assessment, analysis of lab work, and a head-to-toe physical assessment of the patient. Skin care, oral care, pressure ulcer prevention, and urinary catheter maintenance are all involved in the nursing protocol for critically ill patients and are of utmost importance in infection control.

In this chapter you will review:

1. The steps required to complete a head-to-toe assessment.
2. How to provide oral and skin care in the intensive care unit.
3. Pressure ulcer prevention techniques.
4. How to insert a urinary catheter using sterile technique and perform urinary catheter care.

HEAD-TO-TOE ASSESSMENT

A complete head-to-toe assessment is required at the initiation of nursing care to develop and implement the best plan of care. It begins with a patient interview and includes a physical examination, review of all systems, and documentation of IVs, devices, and drains.

A review of a patient's past medical history is also performed and includes interviewing the patient, reviewing the medical record, and speaking with other hospital staff and/or caregivers, as well as, with the patient's family or significant other. It includes previous medical care, surgeries, lab work, and any other pertinent information regarding the patient's health.

Patient Interview

If the patient is stable and able to participate in an interview, introductions should be made, and culturally relevant considerations respected. The patient should state how he or she would like health information released, name a health care proxy, and list specific requests regarding care, religion, and/or culture. **The following issues need to be discussed: chief complaint, history of present illness, past medical history, familial health history, psychosocial history, and available family support, both physical and emotional.**

During the interview, observe the patient's mental status. Note his or her overall appearance, behavior, posture, hygiene, response to questions, clarity of speech, facial expressions, affect, nonverbal indications of pain or discomfort, coordination, orientation to person, place, and time, as well as short- and long-term memory. If the patient is unable to participate in an interview, obtain as much information as possible from the medical record, other health care team members, and the patient's family.

While the patient interview is important, sometimes, especially in critical care, it cannot be completed upon a patient's arrival to the unit. In such cases, acquire pertinent details from other facility staff, the transport team, the rapid-response team, and/or the medical record. Complete a detailed patient interview when and if the patient's condition allows.

Physical Assessment

A complete physical assessment is performed when a patient is admitted to the critical care unit, at least once per shift, and as needed (PRN). It involves all body systems and is very detailed. See Figure 5.1 for general physical assessment guidelines.

Figure 5.1   Example of a General Head-to-Toe Physical Assessment

Neurological System

1. Orientation to person, place, time, and purpose
2. Memory, short- and long-term
3. Affect, attitude, and mood
4. Cognition, speech patterns, and appropriateness of response to questions
5. Pupillary reaction to light, accommodation, and convergence
6. Motor function, balance, coordination, and gait (if possible)
7. Sensory function; note response to pain and tactile stimulation
8. Bilateral hand strength (if possible)

Note: Parts of the neurological system may be assessed during the patient interview.

Head, Eyes, Ears, Nose, and Throat (HEENT)

1. Head: size, shape, symmetry, condition of hair/ scalp, tenderness

Continued

Figure 5.1 *Continued*

2. Eyes:
   a. Symmetry, alignment, and movement
   b. Shape, size, color of pupils
   c. Visual acuity
   d. Peripheral vision
   e. Condition/appearance of conjunctiva and sclera
   f. Condition/appearance of eyelashes, eyebrows, eyelids
3. Ears:
   a. Hearing capability; hearing aids
   b. External ear: shape, size, symmetry, edema, lesions
   c. Ear canal: observe for wax, discharge, foreign bodies
   d. Palpate external ear and surrounding area for pain
4. Nose:
   a. Sense of smell, congestion, difficulty in breathing
   b. Symmetry, drainage, lesions
5. Throat/mouth:
   a. Teeth versus dentures
   b. Condition of lips, gum, tooth, tongue, mucous membrane, uvula, tonsils, hard and soft palate
   c. Color of inside of lip
   d. Lesions, drainage
   e. Odor
   f. Lymph nodes
   g. Trachea/esophagus
   h. Thyroid
   i. Neck veins

Continued

Figure 5.1 *Continued*

Integumentary System

1. History of exposure to caustic materials
2. Any recent skin changes
3. Color
4. Temperature
5. Moisture
6. Areas of redness and/or irritation
7. Breaks in skin: lesions, wounds
8. Scars
9. Bruising, ecchymosis, petechiae
10. Edema
11. Turgor

Respiratory System

1. Question patient regarding:
   a. Shortness of breath
   b. History of respiratory problems
2. Type of O_2 utilized, if any, and delivery appliance
3. Rate, depth, pattern, and number of respirations
4. Oxygen saturation
5. Shape of chest
6. Cough, if applicable
7. Breath sounds; anterior and posterior
8. Palpate chest wall for lumps, pain/tenderness

Cardiovascular System

1. Heart tones; apical pulse, rate, rhythm, and clarity
2. Basic EKG interpretation, if applicable
3. Peripheral pulses; radial, brachial, and pedal
4. Bilateral capillary refill; finger and toe
5. Hemodynamic readings, if applicable

Continued

Figure 5.1   *Continued*

Gastrointestinal/Genitourinary System

1. Question patient regarding
   a. Appetite
   b. Urinary output
   c. Urinary discharge/drainage
   d. Bowel elimination patterns
2. Urine color, clarity, and odor
3. General condition, bulges, scars
4. Assess and evaluate any stomas
5. Auscultate the four quadrants of the abdomen clockwise
6. Palpate the four quadrants for
   a. Distension
   b. Tenderness
   c. Masses
   d. Organ enlargement
   e. Bladder location
7. Assess genitalia and rectal area

Musculoskeletal System

1. Gait (if possible)
2. Bilateral musculature:
   a. Symmetry
   b. Strength and tone
   c. Palpate for lumps, pain/tenderness
3. Joints:
   a. ROM
   b. Pain
   c. Swelling
   d. Crepitation
   e. Nodules

Continued

> **Figure 5.1** *Continued*
>
> 4. Bones:
>   a. Contour
>   b. Prominences
>   c. Symmetry
>
> *Note:* Additional assessment criteria are required for some patient care sets and are detailed in later chapters.

The first step of a physical assessment is to explain to the patient what to expect. **A set of vital signs should be obtained, including temperature, blood pressure, pulse, respirations, and pain. Ask the patient to rate pain on the 1–10 scale, the Wong-Baker Faces, or PAINAD scale.** Nonverbal clues should also be considered to determine the level of pain the patient is experiencing.

IV sites should be documented with notations regarding location, type of device, site appearance, and type of fluid or medication, if any, infusing, along with its corresponding rate. Also include detailed information regarding any type of invasive monitoring equipment (e.g., a PA catheter), drainage system (e.g., a mediastinal chest tube), and/or hemodynamic assistance device (e.g., an IABP).

The steps in a physical assessment can be combined and will become second nature with experience. They can be changed and rearranged to reflect individual patient criteria. **Mini-assessments are made during each shift as nurses implement and evaluate care.**

BASIC PATIENT CARE TECHNIQUES

Oral Care

Oral care for patients in the ICU is important for infection control, good overall health, and patient comfort.

It has been identified by the Centers for Disease Control and Prevention (CDC), the AACN, and the Association for Professionals in Infection Control and Epidemiology (APIC) as a key step in the control and prevention of ventilator-associated pneumonia (VAP). Performing oral interventions decreases dental plaque, helps prevent oropharyngeal bacterial colonization, improves oral cavity hydration, helps prevent reflux, and reduces aspiration of oral secretions.

===*FAST FACTS in a NUTSHELL*

Recommended Nursing Interventions for Oral Care in the ICU

- Elevate the head of the bed at least 30 degrees.
- Brush teeth and gums twice a day with a soft toothbrush.
- Use toothpaste with additives such as sodium bicarbonate.
- Rinse with an alcohol-free, antiseptic mouthwash.
- Floss daily, if possible.
- Suction mouth and oropharnyx PRN.
- Apply water-soluble moisturizer to lips and oral tissues q2h-q4h.
- Avoid lemon-glycerin swabs that may cause excessive drying of oral mucosa.
- Maintain adequate nutritional status.

Skin Care and Pressure Ulcer Prevention

Providing adequate skin care to ICU patients is an important nursing intervention for pressure ulcer prevention, infection control, and patient comfort. Some studies rate the incidence of pressure ulcers in the critical care environment as high as 40%. Skin care protocol starts with a thorough skin assessment, repeated at least every 24 hours, as unit policy dictates, and PRN.

═══════════════════════════*FAST FACTS in a NUTSHELL*

In addition to basic skin care protocol, the following should often be performed:

- Carefully inspect skin for color changes over bony prominences, using a halogen light if needed.
- Compare the texture and temperature of the skin in at-risk areas to surrounding sites: a stage I pressure ulcer may feel stiff, boggy, warmer, or cooler.
- Assess nutritional status; low protein and albumin levels are linked to increased pressure ulcer risk.
- Use a facility-specified skin assessment/pressure ulcer risk tool, such as the Braden Scale.

Once the assessment and corresponding documentation are complete, interventions involving skin care and pressure ulcer prevention are initiated. In the critical care unit, nurses should implement the following steps:

- Use a pressure-redistributing mattress (static air, alternating air, water, or gel).
- Turn the patient q2h, unless contraindicated.
- Do not position the patient directly on their trochanter, unless contraindicated.
- Relieve pressure points q2h.
- Float heels.
- Use proper patient lifting/transferring strategies:
  - Lifting devices such as a trapeze and/or linens.
  - Help from support staff.
- Circulation checks and restraint release q2h, if applicable.
- Consult a dietician to address nutritional issues.

- Complete a daily head-to-toe bath with tepid water and mild soap. Rinse skin well and dry by gentle patting with a towel.
- Use no-rinse soapless bath products when usual bathing techniques are contraindicated.
- Trim nails and wash hair weekly and PRN.
- Apply skin lotion or cream immediately following bath, per hospital policy and/or MD order.
- Use facility-recommended skin protectants.
- Do not massage bony prominences.
- Offer a bedpan/urinal often and with turning/repositioning.
- Provide perineal care during each shift and PRN.
- Implement fecal collectors for loose/liquid bowel movements, while attempting to identify the cause.
- Provide proper colostomy care (refer to facility ostomy department/nurse for hospital specific guidelines, care, and appliances).

(Adapted from Ayello & Sibbald, 2008; Foreman, Milisen, & Fulmer, 2010.)

Range of motion (ROM) exercises are recommended every 4 hours, unless contraindicated, to improve circulation and prevent contracture formation. Record weight daily. As with all procedures and treatments, complete patient education prior to implementation of these measures.

Despite the best efforts of critical care nurses and other health care staff involved in providing proper skin care and preventing pressure ulcers, some patients still develop these painful wounds. When this occurs, **the critical care nurse documents the wound stage, location, size, appearance, and drainage.** He or she should also consult with the hospital wound care department or nurse, who is specially trained to successfully manage pressure ulcers and is an expert in assessment, treatment, facility protocol, and knowledge that can maximize patient comfort while preventing infection.

===============*FAST FACTS in a NUTSHELL*

The Stages of Pressure Ulcers

1. *Stage I*: Non-blanchable erythema; appears as an area of permanent redness in lightly pigmented patients or has a blue/purple appearance in darkly pigmented patients, with a change in skin temperature, edema, and/or hardening of tissue; might be painful or itch.
2. *Stage II*: Blister or abrasion involving dermis and/or epidermis; might appear as a shallow crater.
3. *Stage III*: Ulceration that includes damage to subcutaneous tissue; could extend to, but not through, underlying fascia; appears as a deep crater.
4. *Stage IV*: Deep wound with severe tissue damage, necrosis, and/or involvement of muscle/bone; might exhibit undermining and infection.

(Adapted from Ayello & Sibbald, 2008; Foreman, Milisen, & Fulmer, 2010; Staging Pressure Ulcers, 2010.)

Urinary Catheters

Urinary catheters are inserted for various reasons ranging from the monitoring of the patient's volume status to the resolution of bladder distension to recovery from urologic surgery. In fact, **almost all patients in the ICU have a urinary catheter in place.**

Urinary tract infections (UTIs) account for almost half of all hospital-acquired infections (HAIs). According to the CDC, the cost of treating such HAIs is close to half a billion dollars and 8,000 patient lives a year (2009). Research shows that most hospital-acquired UTIs are related to indwelling urinary catheters. Therefore, **it is extremely important for the critical care nurse to be proficient in the technique of inserting a urinary catheter while maintaining maximum**

sterility. Step-by-step instructions for inserting a urinary catheter using sterile technique are detailed in Figure 5.2.

A bladder scan machine can be used prior to the insertion of a urinary catheter, at the request of a physician

Figure 5.2   How to Insert a Urinary Catheter Using a Sterile Technique

1. Gather supplies:
   a. 14 or 16 Fr urinary catheter for most adults; average length for urinary catheters is 40–45 cm for adults.
   b. Drainage tube and collection bag.
   c. Sterile gloves.
   d. Sterile drapes.
   e. Sterile cotton balls/sponges.
   f. Sterile, disposable forceps.
   g. Sterile povidone-iodine cleansing solution, unless allergic to iodine (confirm alternative protocol with infection control department/MD).
   h. Sterile water-soluble lubricant.
   i. Sterile 10-ml syringe.
   j. Sterile package 10-ml sterile water (or sterile 10-ml pre-filled syringe with sterile water).
   k. 1 amp 2% lidocaine jelly; if ordered for male patient.
   l. Stat-lock tape device; alternately, tape and velcro leg strap.
   m. Disposable underpad.
   n. Extra pad for discarded, used supplies.

Note: At most facilities, items are pre-bundled in a sterile tray-like package.

2. Confirm that the patient has not suffered a urethral injury; review medical history for a possible enlarged prostate.

Continued

Figure 5.2 *Continued*

3. Verify physician's order, assemble supplies at bedside, wash hands.

4. Identify patient via two identifiers such as name, date of birth, and/or medical record number; educate patient regarding procedure.

5. Position patient in a dorsal recumbent position and drape with a sheet, providing as much privacy as possible.

6. Assess perineal area; cleanse, if needed.

7. Place underpad, plastic side down, beneath patient's buttocks.

8. If ordered for a male patient, don gloves and insert approximately 5 ml of 2% lidocaine hydrochloride jelly into tip of penis per facility guidelines.

9. Place extra pad for used supplies on the outer side of the patient's leg, away from where the sterile field will be located.

10. Open drape and/or sterile pack and place between patient's legs.

11. Create a sterile field and open supplies (if packaged separately) in sterile fashion and place on sterile field.

12. Don sterile gloves.

13. Place sterile drape over patient's urethral area.

14. Open povidone-iodine solution and pour over cotton balls/sterile sponges.

15. Open lubricant and apply to urinary catheter tip.

16. Fill 10-ml syringe with sterile water and test catheter balloon.

17. If no leak in balloon, deflate and leave syringe connected.

Continued

Figure 5.2 *Continued*

18. Place the urine specimen cup within easy reach.
19. Cleanse the urinary meatus:
    a. *Female*: Place the thumb and forefinger of nondominant hand between the labia minora, spread, and separate upward. This hand is now **contaminated**. Using the forceps with the remaining sterile hand, pick up a povidone-iodine saturated cotton ball. Swab from above the urinary meatus down toward the rectum, without touching the rectum. Keeping labia separated, clean both labial folds and then directly over the meatus. Never cleanse in an upward manner or go back over a previously cleansed area. Discard each contaminated cotton ball after one downward stroke onto disposal pad. After cleansing the area, drop forceps onto disposal pad. Continue holding labia apart to insert catheter.
    b. *Male*: Grasp the penis between the thumb and forefinger of the nondominant hand. This hand is now **contaminated**. If the patient is uncircumcised, gently retract the foreskin. Use the remaining sterile hand to pick up a povidone-iodine saturated cotton ball with the sterile forceps. Swab from the center of the urinary meatus in an outward circular manner. Continue cleansing outward in larger circles using a new cotton ball for each area. Clean the entire glans. Never go back over a previously cleansed area. Discard each contaminated cotton ball onto

Continued

Figure 5.2 *Continued*

a disposal pad. When cleansing is complete, drop forceps onto disposable pad. Continue holding the penis with the contaminated hand to insert the catheter.

20. Insert and advance the lubricated urinary catheter:
    a. *Female*: Insert the lubricated catheter tip into the urinary meatus, angling the catheter upward as it is advanced; some resistance may be met. Ask the patient to breathe in and out slowly to relax the sphincter muscle. When urine flow is noted, advance the catheter approximately 1 inch further.

Note: If the catheter is unintentionally inserted into the vagina, leave it in place temporarily. Have a staff member obtain another urinary catheter and repeat the entire sterile catheter insertion process. When successful, remove the improperly placed catheter.

    b. *Male*: Hold the penis at a 90-degree angle and insert the lubricated catheter tip into the urinary meatus; some resistance may be met as the catheter is advanced towards the prostatic sphincter. Pause, allowing the sphincter to relax. Lower the penis and advance the catheter into the bladder, where urine will begin to flow.

21. Obtain a sterile urine specimen.
22. Inflate catheter balloon slowly. If balloon will not easily inflate or the patient complains of pain, deflate and advance catheter a nominal amount farther and attempt to reinflate balloon completely.
23. Replace foreskin in an uncircumcised male patient.

Continued

Figure 5.2 *Continued*

24. Remove syringe from catheter.
25. Gently pull catheter downward until there is a feeling of very slight resistance.
26. Attach drainage tube and bag to catheter. Some urinary catheter kits have the tube already attached to the catheter.
27. Secure the stat-lock to the inner aspect of the patient's thigh, allowing for movement and a little slack, without catheter applying pressure, pulling, or shearing at urinary meatus. If a stat-lock type device is not available, use tape and/or velcro leg strap to secure catheter tubing.
28. Secure the drainage bag below the level of the bladder, off the floor, without any dependent loops in the tubing. Never lift a urinary drainage bag above the level of the bladder.
29. Remove drapes and protectors from patient, cleansing the area as needed.
30. Dispose of items properly, remove gloves, and wash hands.
31. Position patient for safety and comfort.
32. Document procedure with date, time, patient reaction, education, and urine amount, color, clarity, and odor.

Note: Never use force to insert a urinary catheter. If continued resistance is met or patient experiences continued pain upon insertion, hold procedure. Seek assistance from charge nurse & physician.

(Adapted from Catheterization, female, 2010; Catheterizing the female & male urinary bladder, 2010; Chenoweth, 2010; Female catheters cause trauma in males, 2010; Heiserman, 2008; Parkland Health & Hospital System, 2009.)

or nurse. It measures the amount of urine in a patient's bladder noninvasively, in just a few minutes. A bladder scan device is extremely easy to use. It is very similar to an ultrasound, can be performed by an RN, and its measurements are accurate. Most hospitals have this machine available and training takes minutes to master.

When providing perineal care for patients with urinary catheters in place, start cleaning from the urinary meatus downward and outward. Do not clean in an upward manner. Use multiple washcloths or perineal cleansing cloths, if needed. Dry promptly. Never use wipes with chlorhexidine solution on the perineal area as it may cause severe irritation.

Review facility specific policies regarding the length of time a urinary catheter can remain in place, when it should be changed, and the protocol regarding proper documentation of physician's orders, insertion, care, and removal of the device.

6

Patient Nutrition

INTRODUCTION

In the critical care unit, patients often have multiple, complex diagnoses. During this time, patient nutrition needs may be overlooked. However, it is precisely within the first 24 to 36 hours of admission when nutritional status should be determined and nutritional supplementation be initiated, if needed.

In this chapter you will learn:

1. The complications caused by malnutrition.
2. How to assess and monitor nutritional status.
3. The basics of enteral and parenteral nutrition.
4. Solutions for common complications encountered with patient nutrition.

THE IMPORTANCE OF NUTRITION IN THE ICU

Reduced food intake, altered digestion, vomiting, diarrhea, trauma, fever, chronic disease, the development of systemic inflammatory response syndrome (SIRS), changes in body composition or serum chemistry, and/or sepsis all cause either a reduction in nutritional intake or an increase in metabolism that can lead to malnutrition. Malnutrition places a patient at high risk for infection, reduced wound healing, the development of a pressure ulcer, poor ventilator weaning, episodes of delirium, impaired organ function, loss of muscle mass, thrombocytopenia, anemia, and lowered immune response. **These risk factors and potential diagnoses can lead to further complications, including an increased length of stay in the hospital or other facility, and a longer recovery and/or rehabilitation time.**

FAST FACTS in a NUTSHELL

The Joint Commission mandates that every patient admitted to a hospital, including those in critical care, receive a nutritional screening.

Although oral intake is the preferred route for patient nutrition, in certain cases, this is simply not possible. Several studies, along with the American Society for Parental and Enteral Nutrition (ASPEN), recommend that some form of nutritional supplementation begin within 36 hours of admission to the hospital or surgery conclusion (Foreman et al., 2010). It is widely accepted that early introduction of nutritional therapy can reduce the risk of infection and improve a patient's overall outcome.

ASSESSING AND MONITORING NUTRITIONAL STATUS

A nutritional assessment is performed as part of the admission assessment. This is accomplished by the completion of a nutritional screening tool. Several different tools exist, with characteristics varying among hospitals, units, and patients to ensure adequate evaluation of specific needs. A nutritional assessment covers various items, including, but not limited to height, weight, body mass index, lab values, an oral health assessment, medication review, past and current nutritional intake status, fluid status, and a determination of current energy requirements.

These assessments are usually completed by an RN but may also be done by the physician and/or dietician. It is important that the patient, family, and multidisciplinary team be involved, including the nurse, doctor, pharmacist, nutritional specialist or registered dietician, and an occupational therapist and/or speech pathologist, if needed.

There is no single way to completely determine a patient's nutritional status. Thus, several tasks are performed to arrive at the best estimate. A dietician or physician often uses a predictive equation that takes into account the patient's minute ventilation, body surface area, age, and temperature, along with various other values to determine an expected energy expenditure. Certain lab tests, such as serum albumin (normal: 3.4–5.4 g/dL), pre-albumin (normal: 15–35 mg/dL), transferrin (normal: >200 mg/dL), hemoglobin (normal: 13–18 for males and 12–16 for females), total lymphocyte count (normal: >1500 mm^3), 24-hour urine creatinine, and 24-hour urine urea nitrogen are indicators of nutritional status.

Nitrogen balance, a determinant that involves monitoring protein intake, is often calculated. Anthropometrical measurements, such as tricep skinfold thickness and midarm circumference, can be measured to estimate nutritional status. Other patient characteristics that are indicators of nutritional status and should be included in daily monitoring are tolerance of enteral feedings, wound healing, presence or absence of infection, serum potassium, magnesium, phosphorus, and the ability to wean from a mechanical ventilator, if applicable.

Oral Nutrition

If a patient in the ICU has a functioning gastrointestinal (GI) system, does not have a nothing by mouth (NPO) order, and is able to tolerate the intake of food and fluids by mouth, the oral route for nutritional intake is preferred. **Patients respond well to oral intake** because they consider it normal and healthy.

Critical care teams should encourage patients to eat and drink at regular mealtimes, as well as when they are hungry or thirsty, providing assistance if necessary. **Several guidelines facilitate positive eating experiences for patients in the ICU:**

- Consult occupational/speech therapists, if needed.
- Keep the room neat and clean, especially during mealtimes, by:
  a. Addressing housekeeping needs prior to mealtime.
  b. Keeping trash cans clean; emptying them often.
  c. Promptly removing dirty linens.
  d. Keeping urinals/bedpans clean; disposing of waste properly.
- Offer toileting and hygiene prior to mealtime.
- Encourage and/or assist with good oral hygiene.
- Allow 30 minutes of rest (i.e., no physical therapy, etc.) prior to meal initiation.
- Reduce distractions during meals.
- Ask visitors to allow patient time to focus on eating.
- Patients experiencing shortness of breath might better tolerate small, frequent meals.
- Provide food and drink portions that reflect the patient's current nutritional needs and appetite.
- Properly position the patient in bed to facilitate comfort during meals and reduce the risk of aspiration.
- Place the food tray and any needed items within the patient's reach.
- Place the call bell within reach.

- Remain present at the bedside, if needed, to assist with meals.
- Allow family/caregiver to remain at the bedside, if needed for assistance.
- Do not rush the patient through meals.
- Educate patient and/or family regarding importance of adequate nutritional intake.

(Adapted from Foreman et al., 2010; Nettina, 2010; Stillwell, 2006; Ukleja et al., 2010.)

If a patient is able to tolerate oral intake yet has additional nutritional needs, **commercially prepared liquid supplements are often initiated**. These "shakes" provide added calories, protein, carbohydrates, fats, vitamins, and minerals. A physician's order is usually required for these oral supplements. It is recommended that a dietician be consulted prior to supplementation.

═══════════════════════════════*FAST FACTS in a NUTSHELL*

Supplemental shakes should be served at room temperature and sipped by the patient. Using the supplement when giving by mouth (PO) medications is a great way to ensure that the patient is actually drinking it, as instructed. Education for the patient and family regarding the importance of these supplement shakes is the key to compliance.

Enteral Nutrition

When a patient is unable to tolerate oral intake related to a physical problem, NPO status, or other reason, nutritional therapy must be initiated. **Enteral nutritional (EN) therapy is the administration of a liquid formula that contains nutrients, such as proteins, carbohydrates, fats, vitamins, and minerals, directly into the stomach, duodenum, or** jejunum via a tube or percutaneous (ostomy) site. There are many types of EN therapy formulas that may provide benefits to specific patient populations based on their ingredients; however, research has not proven that these products are more effective than general EN formulations.

In EN therapy, the formula is started, full-strength, at a minimal rate and increased, as tolerated, to a goal rate that the ordering physician or dietician has specified. "As tolerated" may vary among facilities but normally includes the absence of nausea, abdominal cramping, diarrhea, and high residuals. To be a candidate for EN, a patient must have a functioning GI tract, be hemodynamically stable (i.e., mean arterial pressure >70 mmHg, cardiac index >2.0 l/min/m^2, oxygen saturation >95%), and, if being mechanically ventilated, tolerate a fraction of inspired oxygen (FIO$_2$) <60% with a positive-end-expiratory pressure (PEEP) ≤5 cm.

A tube inserted into the nose, leading to the stomach, duodenum, or jejunum is inserted for patients that require short-term EN. Placement of the tip of the tube into either the duodenum or jejunum is preferred to the stomach because it reduces bowel distension, maintains a better fluid and electrolyte balance, and reduces the risk of aspiration. To prevent aspiration, the jejunum, beyond the ligament of Treitz (Wyckoff et al., 2009), is the best placement for the tip of the tube but can be limited by the skill level of personnel.

An x-ray must be taken and tube placement confirmed by a physician prior to the first use of any type of EN tube that is not inserted surgically (e.g., a percutaneous gastrostomy tube) (PEG). Several bedside techniques for tube placement confirmation exist, such as air auscultation and aspiration of contents for a pH check, but these have been unreliable. For more information about the placement of a feeding tube and EN therapy administration, refer to facility-specific policy and procedure. The *Lippincott Manual of Nursing Practice* is also an excellent resource for procedural information.

======================================*FAST FACTS in a NUTSHELL*

*Several interventions can reduce the risk of
aspiration for patients on EN therapy:*

- Elevate the head of the bed to an angle of at least 30 degrees at all times, unless contraindicated and accompanied by an MD order.
- Use continuous infusion of feeding versus bolus feedings.
- Administer continuous feedings via an electronic controller pump.
- Check residuals every 4 hours.
- Hold feeding and recheck residuals per hospital protocol.
- Discuss administration of metoclopramide with MD to improve gastric motility.
- Closely monitor the patient for abdominal distension.

Complications other than aspiration can arise during EN therapy, such as diarrhea, high residual volume, feeding tube displacement or obstruction, constipation, electrolyte imbalances, azotemia, and serum glucose abnormalities. Tips for preventing and resolving these problems are presented in Figure 6.1. Good oral care is necessary for all patients undergoing EN.

Parenteral Nutrition

Parenteral nutrition (PN), also referred to as total parenteral nutrition (TPN), **is an IV solution made up of a combination of nutritional ingredients** such as water, dextrose, proteins, electrolytes, carbohydrates, lipids, medications (e.g., H2 receptor antagonists and insulin), vitamins, and minerals. PN is initiated when a patient cannot tolerate PO or EN or is

Figure 6.1 Tips for Preventing and Resolving EN Complications

Obstructed Feeding Tube

- Flush tube with 30-ml water q4h.
- Flush tube with 30-ml water before and after medications are given.
- Use medications in liquid form, if possible.
- Finely crush medications that are "crushable" per pharmacy.
- Do not use sugary soda or juice to flush tube.
- If tube becomes obstructed:
  1. Try to flush with 5- to 10-ml warm water.
  2. If tube remains obstructed, attempt to flush with 5- to 10-ml unflavored carbonated soda.
  3. If tube remains obstructed, instill pancre-lipase and sodium bicarbonate per facility policy.
  4. Notify MD if unable to clear obstruction (anticipate tube replacement).

Diarrhea

- Review patient medications noting antibiotics and medications with sorbitol, magnesium, phosphorus, and/or a high osmolarity.
- Avoid use of medications with high sorbitol content.
- Try to give magnesium and/or phosphorus supplements parenterally, if possible.
- Dilute medications with high osmolarity.
- Assess for underlying malabsorption-causing diagnosis and treat as ordered by MD (e.g., pancreatic enzymes).

Continued

Figure 6.1 *Continued*

- Note fiber intake and adjust, PRN.
- Rule out *Clostridium difficile* or treat with antibiotics, if positive.
- Initiate EN therapy at a slow rate, progressing to goal rate as tolerated.
- Use a continuous feeding regimen via a pump.
- Assess for fecal impaction and clear, if necessary.
- Avoid contamination of EN formula:
  1. Maintain aseptic technique when handling formula, tubing, and supplies.
  2. Do not allow formula to hang >8 hours unless ready-to-use container, or facility protocols dictates differently.
  3. Change tubing set q24h or per facility protocol.

Constipation

- Note fiber intake and adjust, PRN.
- Monitor fluid intake and adjust, PRN.
- Review medications for cause, noting antacids with aluminum.
- Administer stool softeners, PRN.
- Encourage activity, if possible.

High Residual Volume

- Minimize narcotics, if possible.
- Assess for and treat any underlying cause of ileus or lowered bowel motility per MD order.
- Monitor serum magnesium and potassium; treat PRN.
- Hold EN therapy and recheck residual in 2 hours or per facility protocol.

Continued

Figure 6.1   *Continued*

- Discuss possible metoclopramide administration with MD.

Electrolyte Imbalances

- Hypokalemia
  1. Monitor and treat blood glucose
  2. Administer supplements, PRN
- Hyperkalemia
  1. Reduced potassium EN formulation for renal-failure patients
  2. Give potassium binders, PRN
- Hyponatremia
  1. Restrict fluid, PRN
- Hypernatremia
  1. Assess for excess water loss
  2. Add water flushes, PRN
- Hypophosphatemia
  1. Monitor blood glucose and treat
  2. Supplement, PRN
- Hypomagnesemia
  1. Assess for signs/symptoms of alcoholism
  2. Supplement, PRN
- Hypermagnesemia
  1. Reduced magnesium EN formula for renal-failure patients
  2. Monitor for and correct acidosis
- Hypocalcemia
  1. Review medications for those that are calcium wasting
  2. Supplement, PRN
  3. Monitor and correct low albumin levels, PRN
  4. Assess Vitamin D intake and supplement, PRN

Continued

Figure 6.1 *Continued*

- Hypercalcemia
  1. Reduced calcium EN formula for renal-failure patients
  2. Encourage ambulation/activity, if possible
  3. Assess vitamin D intake and reduce, PRN

Azotemia

- Reduced protein EN formula, PRN
- Asses for GI bleed

Hypoglycemia

- Monitor blood glucose and adjust insulin doses, PRN
- Remain vigilant about avoiding EN interruptions, if possible

Hyperglycemia

- Monitor blood glucose and administer insulin, PRN
- Assess for signs/symptoms of increased stress and reduce level, if possible
- Assess for signs/symptoms of infection and administer appropriate antibiotics
- Review medications for steroids
- Review medical history for diabetes
- Decrease EN rate, PRN
- Remove dextrose from other sources, if applicable
- Monitor potassium and correct abnormal values, PRN

Continued

Figure 6.1   *Continued*

Note: Some of these guidelines apply for PN, as well. Several interventions require an MD order to complete. Consult with MD, dietician, and additional health care team members prior to implementation.

(Adapted from Foreman et al., 2010; Nettina, 2010; Ross, 2010; Stillwell, 2006, Ukleja et tal., 2010, Wyckoff et al., 2009.)

medically unstable, or if the metabolic demand of the patient is not met via the oral or enteral route.

═══════════════════*FAST FACTS in a NUTSHELL*

PN places the patient at a high risk for infection and costs four to five times more than EN therapy. Thus, EN is preferred over PN when possible because it poses less risk for infection, helps maintain GI function, may prevent hepatic and biliary problems, is generally more nutritionally complete, and costs significantly less.

PN can be administered peripherally (PPN). However, the vein utilized must be large and hold at least a #18 gauge peripheral IV catheter, which is required to handle the high osmolarity of the mixture. PPN contains less than 10% dextrose and is indicated only for patients receiving very short-term therapy.

PN is routinely administered via a central line, with the catheter tip located in the vena cava. Critically ill patients require a PN formulation with at least 10% dextrose and other additives that provide adequate nutrition in correlation with an increased metabolic demand. These mixtures have an increased osmolarity that is beyond the suitability for peripheral administration. The location of the catheter tip should be verified via x-ray prior to PN administration.

A multi-lumen catheter should be used when a patient is receiving PN, with one lumen being dedicated to PN. If this is not possible, PN must be stopped when infusing other fluids and/or medications. The port and lumen line must be flushed with at least 10 ml of normal saline after the PN is stopped, prior to administering the other fluid. After the treatment is complete, the port and lumen is flushed with 10 ml of normal saline. The PN can then be restarted. It should not be infused in the same lumen/line as another IV fluid or medication. Properly clean the central line catheter ports using aseptic technique, according to facility-specific infection control guidelines, prior to access.

A 0.22-µm filter is normally used for PN, but, if it contains lipids, a 1.2-µm filter is used. The filter and tubing should be changed every 24 hours, or per facility protocol.

Patients receiving PN are at higher risk for complications such as infection, bacterial translocation, hypervolemia, hyperosmolar diuresis, pneumonia, gut atrophy, GI bleeding, electrolyte imbalances, and immune system problems than those receiving EN, with the most well-known being catheter-related bloodstream infections. Strict aseptic technique must be used when accessing a patient's central line, completing site care, and performing any activity involving the central line. This helps reduce infection rates. Elevated white blood cell counts and positive blood cultures require administration of the appropriate antibiotics, and typically calls for a central line site change.

Monitoring the patient's lab work and working closely with the health care team to correct abnormalities is the easiest way to prevent complications that can accompany PN therapy. Hyperglycemia is often encountered with PN. It is treated with insulin and the removal of dextrose from other IV fluids, when possible. Electrolyte imbalances can be corrected via changes in the PN formulation and supplements. Elevated liver enzymes can be decreased via alterations in the PN prescription and administration schedule.

Hypervolemia is assessed by daily weight, input/output totals, central venous pressure (CVP), breath sounds, and peripheral edema. It can be controlled with the use of diuretics and the reduction of overall fluid intake. Hyperosmolar diuresis is treated by either lowering the concentration of IV fluids and PN or increasing the total amount of fluid intake. Its presence is determined by reviewing changes in daily weight, input versus output, and CVP.

Encouraging the patient to attempt oral intake and providing ambulation or other activity, if possible, will help reduce the risk for gut atrophy and GI bleeding. Good oral care should be provided to every patient undergoing parenteral therapy.

7

The Sterile Field, Pre-procedural Patient Preparation, and Consciouns Sedation

INTRODUCTION

The critical care environment requires the skills of nurses who are capable of handling any situation, any time, with any number of complications. The procedures of the ICU are as complex as the patients, doctors, and situations that make the unit such a challenging and rewarding place to practice nursing. Aseptic technique, of which a properly prepared and sustained sterile field is an imperative part, must be used during numerous procedures performed at the bedside.

Informed consent and patient education come first when preparing a patient for a procedure, surgery, transfer, or blood transfusion. Because conscious sedation often accompanies many procedures carried out in the ICU, there are strict guidelines for performing this tenuous task while providing a safe environment for the patient.

In this chapter you will learn:

1. The definition of aseptic technique.
2. How to set up and maintain a sterile field.
3. General guidelines for informed consent, pre-procedural patient education and preparation.
4. Guidelines for administration of procedural sedation.

ASEPTIC TECHNIQUE

Surgical site infections remain among the most common nosocomial infections in the United States, despite the technology and infection-control practices currently employed. These potentially lethal infections cause serious complications, result in longer hospital stays, and contribute to the increasing cost of medical care. For these reasons, **it is the responsibility of every nurse to review aseptic technique and sterile field maintenance to improve his or her infection-control practices.**

Aseptic means "without microorganisms," or "germ-free," in layman's terms. **Aseptic technique includes practices for keeping an area, such as a patient's chest, free from pathogens that might cause infection.** It is performed prior to and during surgeries and other procedures. Hand washing, a surgical scrub of the hands and forearms, surgical barriers (e.g., sterile drapes), patient preparation, a sterile field, and the maintenance of a safe environment for the patient and staff are involved in aseptic technique. Many of the steps employed protect both the patient and health care team by preventing contact with pathogens, blood, and body fluids.

When preparing for a sterile procedure, gather all items needed for the procedure prior to the initiation of the sterile prep. **Verify the patient's identity with two patient identifiers and confirm that informed consent has been obtained.** Educate the patient regarding the upcoming sequence of events. If a pre-procedural antibiotic has been ordered, ensure that it has been administered. Often, it is ordered for 30 minutes prior to the procedure or on-call to the operating room. Wash hands with facility-approved "soap" and dry them thoroughly.

Shaving is no longer used in preparing a surgical site. Nicks and abrasions associated with shaving have been proven to be bacterial breeding grounds and possible entrance sites for infection. If needed, clippers can be used to trim hair in the procedural area.

The procedural site must be clean and dry. **Scrub the site and surrounding area with facility-approved antimicrobial soap, generally chlorhexidine or iodophor, in a circular motion.** Begin cleansing at the center and move outward. Use sterile gloves, sponges, and forceps unless other facility guidelines and/or equipment exist.

Wear shoe covers and a surgical cap or hat. All hair must be tucked underneath. Remove jewelry and/or other dangling objects, such as a lanyard holding an I.D. badge. **Wear a facemask and an eye shield (i.e., protective glasses or goggles).**

Members of the health care team who will be participating in the sterile procedure must complete a surgical scrub prior to donning sterile gloves or sterile personal protective equipment (PPE). This is a vigorous forearm-to-fingertip wash, performed for 3–5 minutes with a facility-approved antimicrobial soap. Hands are kept below the elbows while washing to prevent contamination of already cleansed areas. Complete drying is essential to reduce bacteria. Use a sink with a foot pedal, if possible. Do not recontaminate hands by turning off the faucet. Hold hands above elbows once they are dry.

Put on a sterile gown and sterile gloves after the surgical scrub in a clean and/or sterile area, away from the actual sterile field, to lower the risk of contamination. Double gloving is recommended for some procedures to lower the risk of contact with blood and body fluids. Review facility-specific guidelines prior to procedure preparation.

THE STERILE FIELD

Sterile drapes are placed on the patient and on the stand, or tray, that will hold sterile items, equipment, and instruments. Drapes are also placed around the "field" to mark the sterile area. Drapes that establish the sterile field should not be moved once they are in place to lessen the chance of contamination. The outer 1 inch of the sterile field is considered non-sterile.

If possible, a sterile and an unscrubbed team member should be available for procedures to assist the physician(s) and maintain the sterility of the field. Figure 7.1 lists additional guidelines for the set-up and maintenance of a sterile field.

Figure 7.1   Guidelines for the Set-Up and Maintenance of a Sterile Field

- Health care team members with an upper respiratory tract infection and/or cold should not participate in a sterile procedure.
- The front of a sterile gown is sterile from chest level to the level of the sterile field.
- Gown sleeves are sterile from cuffs to 2 inches above elbows, all the way around.
- The back of the gown is **not** sterile; scrubbed team members should never turn their backs toward the sterile field.
- Do not pull gown sleeves up to expose cuffs; sleeves should be long enough to cover the backs of hands.
- Scrubbed team members must keep their hands in front of the body, away from their faces, and above waist level.

Continued

Figure 7.1 *Continued*

- Change contaminated gloves as soon as possible.
- Scrubbed team members must remain close to the sterile field.
- Unscrubbed team members should face the sterile field, not get too close, and never walk between two sterile fields.
- Keep talking to a minimum.
- Do not place sterile products near open windows or doors.
- A sterile tray should be prepared where it will be utilized, as close to use time as possible, and constantly observed for possible contamination.
- When draping, protect gloved hands by cuffing the drape material over the hands.
- Equipment must have a sterile drape on the top, bottom, and sides.
- Only sterile supplies, equipment, etc. should touch a sterile field.
- A sterile drape must cover any stand or equipment immediately next to a sterile field.
- Handle sterile drapes as little as possible to prevent stirring of microscopic particles.
- Apply surgical drapes from the procedural site outward to prevent site contamination.
- Anything below the level of the drapes is considered nonsterile.
- Inspect all items for sterility before dropping them onto the sterile field.
- When dropping items onto a sterile field:
  1. Open the wrapper flap that is farthest away.

Continued

Figure 7.1 *Continued*

2. Open each side flap.
3. Open the nearest flap.
4. Secure all flaps.
5. Offer the item to a scrubbed team member or place onto sterile field.

- Offer sharps and/or heavy items to scrubbed personnel.
- Hand off items to scrubbed team members in a way that prevents a nonsterile person or object from extending over the sterile field.
- Pour solutions into sterile, labeled cups that are placed by a scrubbed person near the edge of the field, not on the "contaminated" portion of the field. Be careful not to splash or spill. Throw away any extra solutions.
- Sterile transfer mechanisms (i.e., a sterile spike or straw) should be employed when dispensing liquid medications.
- When in doubt about the sterility of an item, throw it out.
- Any break in sterility should be corrected immediately, unless contraindicated related to patient safety status.

(Adapted from Alspach, 2006; Aseptic technique and the sterile field, 2005; Hauswirth & Sherk, 2010; Infection, asepsis, and sterile techniques, 2010; Introduction to sterile technique, 2010; Nettina, 2010; Recommended practices for maintaining a sterile field, 2006.)

INFORMED CONSENT

Informed consent must be obtained from a patient prior to a procedure, surgery, facility transfer, experimental/investigational treatment, or blood-product administration.

It is considered an agreement between the patient and the physician based on a conversation that has transpired.

══════════════════════════════*FAST FACTS in a NUTSHELL*

In the conversation that constitutes informed consent, the physician and patient discuss:

- Exactly who will be performing the procedure; the physician's identity.
- The specific nature of the planned procedure.
- The benefits and risks of the procedure.
- Alternative treatments available.
- Pain control and/or anesthesia during the procedure.

The discussion occurs prior to the administration of any sedative medications. Afterwards, when all of the patient's questions have been answered, an informed consent form is signed. **The form verifies that the conversation between the physician and patient took place and that both are in agreement about the procedure.** A nurse may serve as a witness to the signatures.

If the patient is unable to provide consent because of physical and/or mental incapacity, a legal guardian, health care proxy, or the next of kin can provide consent. Ideally, the patient has a living will or a designated health care proxy. If not, the general order for persons who can give consent for treatment is:

1. A spouse, including common law
2. An adult child
3. A parent
4. A sibling
5. A surrogate

If no relative or guardian is available, two physicians can indicate that the procedure must be completed due to a dire risk to the patient's health.

These guidelines change slightly when a minor is involved. Verification of specific facility protocol is important. If the patient is unable to give consent, the reason must be documented.

Several things should be clear on the informed consent form:

- Patient identity
- The procedure, surgery, blood product, etc. to be completed:
  a. In layman's terms, if possible
  b. No abbreviations
- Name of actual physician performing the procedure
- Statement that alternatives have been discussed
- Statement that benefits, risks, and possible side effects have been discussed
- Pain control and/or anesthesia authorization
- Disposition of specimens or body parts, if applicable
- Any special circumstances or considerations
- Signature of patient, or person, providing consent, noting time and date
- Signature of physician who obtained the consent, noting time and date
- Signature of person witnessing patient's/proxy's signature, noting time and date

FAST FACTS in a NUTSHELL

Informed consent should be obtained for a patient's refusal of treatment, including blood products. The release and electronic transmission of medical records also requires documented informed consent.

PRE-PROCEDURAL PATIENT PREPARATION

Patient Education

Patient education is a major part of nursing care. In the ICU, it occurs throughout a shift and may apply to the family as much as to the patient. When possible, education regarding pre-procedural events, the actual procedure, and post-operative expectations, activities (e.g., incentive spirometry use), and recovery should be provided.

Education is best provided at the patient's and/or family's level of understanding in multiple ways, such as verbal, demonstrative, and audiovisual techniques. The following elements should be included in pre-procedural patient education:

- Cultural/religious considerations
- Interpreters, chaplains, other health care team members as needed
- Family/significant others, if possible
- Explanation of pre-op events
- How the procedure/test/medications may make the patient feel
- Description of immediate post-op environment and any involved equipment (e.g., ventilator, chest tubes)
- Approximate starting time of procedure
- Approximate length of procedure
- Location of visitor waiting area
- Visiting hours
- Projected length of stay and expected follow-up
- Patient/family responsibilities regarding post-op care and recovery

Basic Patient Preparation

Patients should be prepared for a procedure, surgery, blood-product administration, or other procedural activity according to facility-specific guidelines. However, some basic preparation steps are completed before most procedures, such as:

- Verification of patient identity with two patient identifiers
- Verification of informed consent completion

- Verification of drug allergies
- Administration of pre-op or on-call medication(s)
- Verification that the correct site has been marked, if applicable
- Verification of NPO status
- Gown is in place, without additional clothing items
- Proper skin prep is complete, if applicable
- Dentures, bridges, and/or partials are removed, put in a labeled cup, and stored properly
- Glasses or contacts are removed and properly stored
- Jewelry is removed and secured per facility policy
- The patient has voided or a urinary catheter is in place, if ordered

Procedural Sedation

There are three definitions of *procedural sedation:*

1. *Minimal-drug-induced state:* Thinking and motor function may decrease but patient responds to verbal commands. Respiratory and cardiovascular (CV) functions are not impaired.
2. *Moderate-drug-induced state:* Thinking and motor function decrease. Patient may respond to verbal commands, or verbal commands with light tactile stimulation may be required to elicit a response. Respiratory and CV functions should be unaltered. This is often referred to as conscious sedation.
3. *Deep-drug-induced state:* The patient requires either painful stimulation or multiple stimulation attempts to be aroused. The airway may become compromised; however, CV function should be unaltered. This is considered monitored anesthesia and is administered by a physician or certified registered nurse anesthetist (CRNA).

How and by whom procedural sedation is administered varies among states and facilities. Several state boards of nursing (SBNs) have guidelines addressing this practice, while others do not. Clarification can be obtained from the SBN and facility where the procedure will be occurring.

Several bedside procedures, such as insertion of a central line or chest tube, involve a nurse inducing moderate conscious sedation. A physician will also be present. Several key components must be addressed prior to the initiation of moderate sedation:

1. A pre-procedural assessment must be performed noting:
   a. Baseline vital signs, including oxygen saturation
   b. Drug allergies
   c. Airway assessment
   d. History of respiratory system problems or airway-related difficulties
   e. Previous difficulties with sedation/anesthesia
   f. Last time of oral intake and what was consumed
   g. Current medication list
   h. History of alcohol or drug use
   i. Pain
   j. Pregnancy status
   k. Organ system abnormalities
2. Verification of two patient identifiers
3. Verification of signed informed consent
4. Patient/family education
5. Oxygen: nasal cannula and facemask
6. Availability of emergency supplies at bedside:
   a. Suction supplies and working suction equipment
   b. Artificial airways: oralpharyngeal and nasopharyngeal airways in proper sizes
   c. Crash cart and defibrillator
7. Ordered sedation medications in proper doses at bedside
8. Reversal medications in proper doses at bedside
9. Patent IV
10. Procedure/site verification and completion of a "time-out"

(Adapted from Alspach, 2006; Consent Titles for Cath Lab Patients, 2010; Nettina, 2010.)

During the procedure, care must be taken to monitor the patient's respiratory status and vital signs. Hemodynamic monitoring should also be performed, if applicable. Frequent sedation assessments should be performed per facility policy and documented via a sedation scale such as the Ramsay Assessment Scale for Adult Patients or the Richmond Agitation-Sedation Scale. Such scales rate patient response, sedation, agitation, and motor activity. Medications should be titrated to the desired effect for each patient while maintaining adequate vital signs and a patent airway. Once the procedure is finished and sedation is no longer required, monitoring of the patient should continue per facility protocol with the appropriate documentation completed.

=====*FAST FACTS in a NUTSHELL*

Several medications can be used during moderate sedation, such as diazepam (Valium), midazolam (Versed), fentanyl (Sublimaze), morphine, merperidine (Demerol), and, occasionally, ketorolac (Toradol). Naloxone (Narcan) and flumazenil (Romazicon) are both reversal drugs that are to be kept at the bedside during procedural sedation. The physician might also order other medications to be given.

All medications should be verified prior to administration. Not all SBNs and/or facilities allow registered nurses to manage the drugs discussed.

Sedation, other than procedural, is frequently required in the ICU for patient anxiety, agitation, pain, and/or delirium. It is important to address assessments, medications, and emergency preparations with the same concern as if the patient were undergoing procedural sedation. Similar sedation scales are used, and the medications are often the same. Pain and delirium should be assessed using a facility-approved scale.

8

Isolation Precautions and Personal Protective Equipment

INTRODUCTION

The critical care unit is home to a diverse group of patients suffering from any number of medical issues, including infection. These patients are also immunocompromised as a result of their underlying disease processes, placing them at high risk for a nosocomial infection. Studies have shown that while the ICU makes up a small number of the beds in most facilities, 20% of hospital-acquired infections (HAIs) occur there. Patients with burns involving >30% total body surface area are at the greatest risk for HAIs.

This information leads to a discussion of two extremely important topics: isolation precautions and personal protective equipment (PPE). Use of these valuable instruments is vital to protect health care workers and patients from potential infections, such as tuberculosis, C. difficile, hepatitis, and Staphylococcus aureus (S. aureus).

In this chapter you will learn:

1. The types of isolation precautions and their corresponding guidelines.
2. The types of PPE, along with usage guidelines.
3. Needle-stick prevention.

ISOLATION PRECAUTIONS

Protecting patients and health care workers from the transmission of infection requires vigilance on the part of the entire medical community, from the facility administration to the janitorial staff. The Joint Commission has issued guidelines, called Standard and Transmission-Based Isolation Precautions, for facilities to follow to help meet patient safety goals related to infection prevention. The World Health Organization (WHO) issued an initiative called Hand Hygiene in Health Care, which is a major component of every precaution modality. Both involve numerous steps, supplies, and equipment.

Health care facilities are charged with the education and training of their staff regarding infection-control practices. They are also responsible for providing the equipment and engineering controls needed to comply with such practices.

Studies have shown that **precaution adherence improves with adequate nurse-patient staffing ratios.** Facilities are encouraged to engage enough nurses and support personnel to allow for maximum compliance. With education, training, support, supplies, and equipment, it is then up to the staff to implement the precautions and use the proper PPE.

Several types of pathogens cause infection, including bacteria, viruses, fungi, parasites, and prions. These infectious organisms are transmitted via the following routes:

- Contact, direct or indirect
- Droplet

- Airborne
- Blood borne

Contact is the most common way a pathogen is transmitted. This route is further divided into two forms: direct and indirect.

Direct contact occurs when a microorganism is transmitted from one person to another without an intermediary. Indirect contact occurs when a pathogen is transmitted to a person from a contaminated article or person. For example, a patient can be infected with *C. difficile* from contact with the contaminated hands of a nurse who cared for a pathogenic patient but is not infected.

Droplet transmission occurs when respiratory droplets >5 micrometers, traveling short distances, contain infectious microorganisms, such as the influenza virus. The droplets are not pathogenic past approximately 3 feet.

These droplets are produced in various ways, for example, when the host coughs, sneezes, talks, is suctioned, or is intubated. The droplets may come into direct contact with the mucosal tissue of another viable host or may be transferred by other direct or indirect contact.

Airborne transmission involves fine airborne particles that contain pathogens. These particles remain infectious over long distances and for a longer period of time than do larger droplets. Tuberculosis is transmitted in this fashion.

Blood-borne transmission occurs when blood that contains pathogens comes in contact with susceptible tissue, for example, when a nurse is stuck with a contaminated needle. Hepatitis B is a blood-borne disease.

Precautions are based on the mode of transmission of the potential pathogen. There are two types of precautions:

- Standard: Implemented for every patient
- Transmission-based: Based on the presumed pathogenic organism

Transmission-Based Precautions are taken in addition to Standard Precautions and hand hygiene.

===============*FAST FACTS in a NUTSHELL*

Isolation precautions is technically an outdated term, with the Centers for Disease Control and Prevention (CDC) currently using *precautions to prevent transmission of infectious agents* (2007).

Transmission-Based Precautions should be instituted at the time the patient exhibits symptoms that indicate a potential infection, because lab identification and/or confirmation of microorganisms can take several days. Consultation with the facility's infection-control nurse or other specified personnel should occur as soon as possible.

Hand hygiene is necessary for all facility staff, patients, family members, and visitors. This includes hand washing and, when hands are not visibly soiled, using alcohol-based hand-cleansing products.

STANDARD PRECAUTIONS

Standard Precautions are executed for each and every patient. According to the CDC, "Standard Precautions constitutes the primary strategy for the prevention of health care associated transmission of infectious agents among patients and health care personnel." (2007). This is an impressive statement and is echoed by several other associations.

It is important to understand and employ Standard Precautions in every nursing interaction. **Gloves, a gown, mask, and eye protection are worn, depending on the level of exposure to blood, body fluids, secretions, and excretions.** Respiratory Hygiene/Cough Etiquette, safe injection practices, and the use of masks during procedures involving a lumbar puncture are also included in Standard Precautions.

According to Standard Precautions guidelines, hand hygiene should be completed after contact with any blood, body fluid, secretion, excretion, or potentially contaminated object; immediately after taking off gloves; and between patient contacts.

Gloves should be worn when there is the risk of contact with blood, body fluids, secretions, excretions, contaminated objects, mucous membranes and/or nonintact skin.

A protective, facility-approved gown should be worn when there is risk of contact between clothing and/or exposed skin and blood, body fluids, secretions, and excretions.

A mask, eye protection, and/or a face shield should be worn during tasks with the potential for splashes and sprays of blood, body fluids, and/or secretions. Suctioning and intubation are high-risk processes for exposure to respiratory secretions; therefore, it is strongly suggested that a mask and eye protection be worn during these procedures.

═══════════════════════════════*FAST FACTS in a NUTSHELL*

Important aspects of Standard Precautions involve equipment and the facility environment. Recommendations include:

- Handle soiled equipment such that it does not contaminate the environment, personnel, or other patients.
- Disinfect equipment according to manufacturer guidelines.
- Disinfect computers, phones, etc. used in patient care areas per facility policy.
- Remove soiled laundry properly. Avoid shaking it; do not allow it to contact clothing or body, and place it in a laundry bag.
- Disinfect surfaces in patient care areas per facility policy, with EPA-registered cleansers.

Needle-stick prevention is a component of Standard Precautions that protects the nurse from exposure to blood-borne pathogens. Engineering controls and safety devices should be used if possible. Examples of prevention products include retractable needles, protective sheaths, shielded IV catheters, needleless injection systems, and plastic blood-collection tubes. Do not recap, bend, or break needles. Always use puncture-proof sharp containers.

═══════════════════════════════*FAST FACTS in a NUTSHELL*

Part of Standard Precautions is protecting patients with safe injection practices:

- The use of sterile, single-use, disposable needles and syringes
- The use of single-dose medication vials
- The use of aseptic technique for all injections

Some infection-control issues are related to lumbar punctures. To help combat these issues, The Health Care Infection Control Practices Advisory Committee recommends that **any professionals accessing the spinal or epidural space wear a mask** (CDC, 2007).

Respiratory Hygiene/Cough Etiquette is also a component of Standard Precautions and applies to anyone with signs of sickness such as cough, congestion, nasal drainage, and/or respiratory secretions who enters a health care facility. Implementation includes:

- Educating health care workers, patients, family, and visitors.
- Posting signs, in various languages, detailing guidelines.
- The proper use and disposal of tissues for nasal drainage, sneezing, and coughing.
- Wearing of masks for persons with a cough, if applicable.
- Proper hand hygiene.
- Spatial separation of >3 feet, when possible, for persons with suspected respiratory infections.

CONTACT PRECAUTIONS

Contact precautions are implemented when caring for a patient who is suspected of having an infectious agent, such as diarrhea or an abscessed wound, **that is spread by either direct or indirect contact.** Contact precautions, in addition to Standard Precautions, include:

- A single-patient room, if possible
- Wearing gloves and a gown when entering the patient's room
- Wearing other task-related PPE when entering the patient's room and discarding all prior to leaving

DROPLET PRECAUTIONS

Droplet precautions are practiced when a patient is suspected of having an infectious agent, such as influenza, *Neisseria meningitis,* or the mumps, **that is spread through droplet transmission.** Droplet precautions, in addition to Standard Precautions, include:

- A single-patient room, if possible
- Wearing a mask when entering the patient's room, related to potential close patient contact
- If transported out of his or her room, the patient wears a mask

AIRBORNE PRECAUTIONS

Airborne precautions are taken when a patient exhibits symptoms related to an infection, such as tuberculosis (TB) or severe acute respiratory syndrome (SARS), that **is transmitted over long distances and suspended in air.** Airborne precautions, in addition to Standard Precautions, include

- Housing patients in an airborne-isolation room, such as a negative-pressure room with 6–12 air exchanges per hour and exhaust directed outside the building or through high-efficiency particulate air (HEPA) filtration before it is returned.

- A respirator or a mask with N95 or higher rating must be in place before entering the patient's room

(Adapted from Siegel et al., 2007.)

PERSONAL PROTECTIVE EQUIPMENT

PPE **is a vital component of infection-control and isolation precautions.** Proper use of such equipment protects the health care team, patients, family members, and visitors.

Isolation precautions apply to facility staff, patients, family members, and visitors.

Signs indicating the type of Transmission-Based Precautions required to enter the patient's room should be posted clearly outside the patient's room along with instructions on how to properly apply PPE. The equipment and supplies needed should be available near the entrance to the patient's room.

Gloves

Gloves are an integral part of PPE and come in a variety of materials, including latex, nitrile, and vinyl. **Choosing the proper glove is important.** It is based on individual preference, the expected contact with chemicals, latex sensitivity, size, and facility policy. Gloves should be powder-free.

Because patient care starts in clean areas and moves to potentially contaminated areas, a change of gloves may be required. Gloves must also be changed and hand hygiene performed when facility personnel move from one patient to another.

When donning gloves and other PPE, gloves are put on last. They should fit snugly at the wrist and cover the gown cuff, if applicable.

Gloves are disposable, not reusable. Remove a glove by grasping it near the wrist and peeling downward. The glove should be taken off inside out and held inside the remaining gloved hand. Slide the index finger under the wrist of the remaining glove and peel it downward. The initial glove should be contained in the second glove, which will be inside out. Throw gloves into the proper waste receptacle.

Isolation Gown

An isolation gown is a component of PPE whose use is dictated by the precaution instituted, the Occupational Safety and Health Association (OSHA) Blood Borne Pathogens Standard, and the task to be completed. **An isolation gown protects the arms, body, and clothing from being exposed to possible pathogens.** The gown is always worn with gloves and should be put on before any other PPE. Gloves should cover the gown cuff when applied.

The proper method of removing a gown prevents contamination. A gown should be removed before leaving the patient's room. After removing gloves, goggles or a face shield, and mask, if applicable, untie the gown and peel it down from the neck and shoulders, turning the contaminated outer side inward. Roll it into a bundle and throw it in the proper waste receptacle.

Mask, Goggles, and Face Shield

A mask, goggles, and/or face shield are worn when:

- Indicated by a Transmission-Based isolation precaution.
- The potential for a blood or body fluid spray/splash exists.
- The potential for respiratory secretion exposure exists.
- Aseptic technique is performed.
- Staff members feel that it is necessary.

These items protect the eyes, nose, and mouths of the health care team while protecting the patient from possible exposure to pathogens from the team. OSHA also mandates the use of these items.

Masks, goggles, and face shields come in a variety of sizes, shapes, combinations, and materials. **Product selection is based on the task to be completed, facility specifications, and individual preference.** Eyeglasses are not considered sufficient protection and should be supplemented.

Facial protection is put on after an isolation gown and before gloves, when applicable. Goggles and/or a face shield are removed before the gown and properly disposed of. A mask or respirator is removed after the gown, before hand hygiene.

Unless clearly labeled, a mask or face shield is not to be considered a respirator, or N95 mask. OSHA has multiple mandates applicable to these types of masks. For example, every staff member must be fit-tested for a facility-approved respirator, or N95 mask, prior to participating in airborne precautions. This equipment is donned in the same fashion as a mask when wearing additional PPE. **It is applied before entering an airborne-precaution area.** A respirator, or N95 mask, should be removed after an isolation gown.

═══════════════════════════════════*FAST FACTS in a NUTSHELL*

More tips for minimizing exposure to pathogens include:

- Avoid touching one's own mouth, nose, eyes, and face while working.
- Position patients in a way that directs possible splashes/sprays away from staff.
- Always put on PPE properly.
- Remain current with immunizations, such as a flu shot.
- Complete hand hygiene after removing PPE and frequently throughout the day. Encourage others to do so.

Patients for whom Transmission-Based Precautions are taken may suffer from anxiety and depression related to the stigma associated with the precautions and the possibility of reduced interaction with staff, family, and visitors. **Adequate education and emotional support, along with nonjudgmental interaction, will help improve these outcomes.**

9

Everything IV

INTRODUCTION

Medication and fluid delivery are important aspects of critical care nursing, although many obstacles make performing these tasks difficult. If a patient is intubated, unconscious, or otherwise unable to tolerate oral (PO) intake, another means to provide hydration and medication must be used. The most effective route to introduce medication and fluids is through intravenous (IV) access, such as a peripheral IV (PIV) inserted in a forearm, a peripherally inserted central catheter (PICC), or a central venous line (CVL).

Intravenous fluid therapy is utilized in various ways to accomplish medical treatments. These solutions have distinct characteristics that achieve desired outcomes such as hydration, volume expansion, and increased blood pressure.

Patient-controlled analgesia (PCA) is a fantastic way to manage pain in the ICU; however, it requires a participating patient along with a vigilant, well-educated nurse.

Critical care nurses are well versed in the types of IVs, corresponding insertion procedures, and maintenance techniques. They also understand how IV therapy is used as a tool for patient treatment.

In this chapter you will learn:

1. The basics of IV therapy.
2. How to properly insert, assess, and maintain a PIV.
3. How to maintain and monitor a PICC and other types of CVLs.
4. How to administer medication through an IV access site.
5. The ins and outs of PCA.

THE BASICS OF IV THERAPY

IV therapy is initiated for various reasons, including fluid and electrolyte maintenance, the administration of medication, blood products, diagnostic reagents (e.g., for contrast during a CT scan), nutrition, and hemodynamic monitoring. The access site can be peripheral or central.

========================*FAST FACTS in a NUTSHELL*

IV therapy is based on the principles of osmosis, diffusion, and filtration. IV fluids are classified into three main categories: hypertonic, hypotonic, and isotonic. They can also be either crystalloids or colloids. The category assigned to an IV solution is based on its composition and affect on body cells.

Hypotonic solutions hydrate the cells of the body. Commonly used types are ½ normal saline (NS) and ¼ NS. This therapy is used for patients who require dialysis or diuretic therapy, or who are in diabetic ketoacidosis. Patients with increased intracranial pressure or burns should not receive hypotonic fluids.

Hypertonic solutions pull fluid out of the cells, increasing intravascular volume. Included in this category of solutions are 5% dextrose (D5) NS, D5 0.45% NS, saline 3%, albumin 25%, and total parenteral nutrition (TPN). These IV fluids help stabilize blood pressure and can increase urine output. Close monitoring must be used when infusing these therapies, as intravascular volume overload and pulmonary edema can occur.

Isotonic solutions do not cause a change in cellular hydration. Examples of these types of IV fluids are lactated ringer's (LR), D5 in water (W), 0.9% NS, plasma, and albumin 5%. Patients should be monitored for symptoms associated with circulatory overload when receiving such therapy.

IV solutions can be colloids or crystalloids. Colloids contain macromolecules and, often, protein. Blood, human albumin, and hespan are frequently used colloids. These fluids can cause major fluid shifts, especially in critically ill patients.

NS, LR, and several of the dextrose combinations are crystalloid solutions. These IV fluids are full of small solutes, which are efficient volume expanders, and can be used to provide fluid replacement.

FAST FACTS in a NUTSHELL

Several precautions regarding IV therapy include:

- D5W: Is used to replace water loss; is a carrier for several medications:
  - Cannot be infused with blood or blood products.
  - Not given to patients with water intoxication.
- NS: Is used to replace saline loss, given with blood products, and can be used to treat hemodynamic shock:
  - Not given to patients with isotonic volume excess.
  - Monitor for fluid overload.
- LR: Is used to replace isotonic fluid loss, frequently given after surgery, and can replenish minimal electrolyte loss and correct mild metabolic acidosis:
  - Not given to patients with alkalosis or liver disease.

PERIPHERAL IV

IV therapy is frequently performed via a peripheral IV (PIV) catheter. PIVs are commonly placed in the hand, forearm, and upper arm, where adequate veins, such as the dorsal, ascendens, basilic, cephalic, and cubital, are located. A nurse normally performs the insertion, and even though it is considered a basic procedure, **aseptic technique must be used.** Sterile gloves are not required, but the area should be cleansed with chlorhexidine, or as facility policy dictates, prior to needle insertion.

Tips for achieving and maintaining a successful PIV include:

- Verify the physician's order.
- Confirm any patient allergies. If allergic to plastic tape, apply paper or cloth tape.
- Choose the appropriate catheter/needle gauge for the selected vein.
- Explain the procedure to the patient and obtain verbal consent.
- Wear gloves throughout PIV insertion.
- Administer a Xylocaine wheel of 1% prior to PIV insertion, if facility policy, nurse discretion, and patient consent allow.
- Apply a tourniquet 2–6 inches above the intended insertion site for best vein visualization.
- Use the same finger of the nondominant hand to palpate the vein for every PIV attempt.
- Avoid veins that feel cordlike and hard.
- Insert the needle bevel up.
- A nurse is allowed only two attempts at obtaining access.
- Do not reinsert a catheter stylet back into a catheter.
- Observe for blood flashback.
- Secure PIV with tape and/or facility-approved bio-occlusive dressing.
- Label the site with date, time, gauge, and initials.

- If administering IV fluids, secure tubing and catheter connections well.
- Assess PIV site every 4 hours.
- Change dressing every 3 days and PRN.
- Rotate PIV site every 72 hours.

(Adapted from Alexander, 2006; Hadaway, 2007; Lee, 2009; Nettina, 2010.)

CENTRAL VENOUS LINES

Peripherally Inserted Central Catheter

A physician, radiologist, advanced practice nurse, or specially trained RN can insert a peripherally inserted central catheter (PICC). **The procedure is sterile** and may take place at the bedside, in the OR, or in a technical room. Single- or multi-lumen catheters are available and capable of long-term IV therapy. Some brands are able to withstand pressure from CT injections (check manufacturer guidelines).

A PICC is inserted in the basilic, median cubital, or cephalic vein, usually guided by ultrasound. The tip is advanced to a site located between the lower one-third of the superior vena cava (SVC) to the junction of the SVC itself, and the right atrium. A chest x-ray is taken to confirm placement. If the tip is located in the subclavian or innominate vein, the physician may still approve catheter use. However, hyperalimentation would be contraindicated.

Verification and application of facility policies regarding infusions and care is necessary. A few guidelines of importance regarding PICCs include:

- Do not take blood pressure in the arm where the PICC is located.
- Document the catheter's location and length protruding from the insertion site.
- Confirm that the length line has not changed with each assessment and medication administration.

- Always use a 10-ml syringe to access a PICC.
- Waste at least 5-ml of blood prior to each blood draw.
- Flush turbulently with 10-ml NS every shift and before and after blood draws, intermittent infusions, medications, TPN, etc.
- Change all caps weekly and with all blood draws, using aseptic technique.
- Use aseptic technique during site care.
- Initial dressing change should occur 24 hours after PICC insertion.
- Change dressing every 7 days and PRN.
- Cover with a bio-occlusive dressing only, no 4 × 4s.
- Never attempt to reinsert or remove a partially dislodged PICC. Secure it with steri-strips, cover with sterile 4 × 4s and kling wrap. Notify the physician immediately.

Other Central Venous Catheters

There are other types of CVLs. The location, style, and access for medication administration vary among the types of catheter utilized. Often referred to as central venous access devices (VADs), their care is similar to that of a PICC. Major differences are noted below.

A midline catheter is not actually a CVL. It is technically a "deep peripheral" IV site, located in the basilic, cephalic, or median cubital vein. The interior tip should rest at the distal to axillary arch. Hyperalimentation and certain antibiotics cannot be infused through this site.

Implanted ports are true CVLs. The port is inserted surgically into the chest wall. There are no real visible signs of the device exteriorly except a small, palpable bulge. One or two small pliable nodules indicate the core of the device, surrounded by a harder rim. The internal tip of the catheter should rest in the SVC.

Ports are accessed with a noncoring Huber needle, using aseptic technique. If possible, apply lidocaine/prilocaine (EMLA) topically to the skin around the port prior to access.

This will improve patient comfort during the procedure. Blood aspiration should be performed prior to administering anything through the port. If aspiration is unsuccessful, call the physician. Anticipate a chest x-ray to confirm placement.

Dressings are changed every 7 days, when the needle is changed (at least every 7 days), and PRN. A 5-ml heparin flush may be indicated at some facilities; confirm policy prior to administration.

A tunneled catheter is similar to a PICC, but is "tunneled" under the skin of the chest wall into a central vein, frequently the subclavian. The interior tip should rest in the SVC. Approximately 4 inches of the catheter extends out of the skin. The end is closed with a needleless luer lock cap. This procedure is done in the operating room (OR).

Common types of tunneled catheters are the Groshong, Hickman, and Broviac. **Physician preference, along with facility supply, dictates which type of tunneled catheter is inserted.** The catheter may be single- or multi-lumen.

The Hickman and Broviac have a Dacron cuff located approximately 1 inch from the exit site into the skin that helps maintain catheter placement and provides a barrier against infection. The Groshong contains a three-way valve and does not require clamping.

Dressings are changed daily for 1 week post-insertion, then every 3 days until the site is healed. No further dressings are normally required. The exposed catheter should be secured to the chest wall with tape.

In the ICU, another type of VAD, called a Cordis or introducer, is employed for hemodynamic monitoring and usually inserted in the right internal jugular. It is a large, thick, single lumen sheath with access for a PA catheter. It has a small tubing arm, allowing IV access, on the side. Dressings are changed every 72 hours and PRN. PA catheters and hemodynamic monitoring are discussed in Chapter 11.

A double- or triple-lumen percutaneous CVL is also regularly used in critical care. The internal jugular or subclavian vein is the most common access site; however, the femoral is sometimes used. These lines are used to monitor central venous pressure (CVP), perform transvenous pacing, draw blood, and administer fluid, medications, and/or parental nutrition. Dressings are changed at 72-hour intervals and PRN.

FAST FACTS in a NUTSHELL

Implementations for central lines involve flushing, frequent assessment, and dressing changes. Most of these devices are negative pressure and must be clamped when not in use. A few other CVLs are available and require similar care. After identifying the catheter type, refer to facility policy/procedure for specifications.

When preparing for, and assisting with, the insertion of a CVL, several guidelines should be followed:

- Confirm consent.
- Confirm patient identity via two patient identifiers.
- Educate patient/family and provide emotional support
- Clip hair located at the insertion site; do not shave.
- Use aseptic technique during catheter changes over a guide wire. Caps, masks, eye protection, sterile gowns, and large sterile drapes are used.
- Place the patient in Trendelenburg position for a subclavian or jugular insertion.
- After site preparation, sterile gloves are changed prior to insertion of the actual central venous access device.
- During PA catheter insertion, the physician or advanced practice nurse must change sterile gloves after introducer insertion, before the PA catheter is placed. An additional sterile field should also be introduced at this time.
- Ensure placement of a sterile, occlusive dressing over the site.

- Auscultate bilateral breath sounds, post-insertion.
- Confirm that a chest x-ray has been performed and read, post-insertion, before administering fluids or medications.

(Adapted from Alexander, 2007; Chohan & Munden, 2007; Ehlers, 2007; Lee, 2009; Nettina, 2010; Stillwell, 2006; Wyckoff et al., 2009.)

Discontinuing and Removing a VAD

An RN can discontinue some VADs at the bedside, when ordered. There are several steps to follow:

1. Confirm the order.
2. Verify patient identity via two patient identifiers.
3. Educate patient/family and provide emotional support.
4. If catheter is located in neck, place the patient in Trendelenburg position.
5. Ask the patient to turn head away from site, if applicable.
6. Remove and properly dispose of dressing.
7. Remove any sutures using aseptic technique.
8. If the tip of the VAD is to be cultured, don sterile gloves, mask, and cap.
9. Smoothly and swiftly pull the catheter back until tip is removed from skin.
10. If any resistance is met, stop. The catheter should not be forcibly removed. Leave it in place, cover site with sterile 4 × 4, and notify the physician.
11. Apply pressure to site until hemostasis is attained.
12. Note that the catheter tip is intact and discard properly, unless culture of tip is to be obtained.
13. Place a sterile occlusive dressing on the site.
14. Document procedure, site appearance, catheter length and appearance, and patient tolerance.
15. Change dressing every 24 hours and PRN, assessing site until healed.

(Adapted from Alexander, 2007; Chohan & Munden, 2007; Ehlers, 2007; Lee, 2009; Nettina, 2010; Stillwell, 2006; Wyckoff et al., 2009.)

A physician, physician's assistant, advance practice nurse, or specially trained RN removes tunneled catheters and implantable ports, often in the OR.

COMPLICATIONS OF IV THERAPY

Potential complications arising from IV therapy are numerous. They can result from the insertion of the device, the therapy, or the IV access device itself. **Most complications can be prevented** by closely monitoring the patient for changes, proper device insertion, and adherence to aseptic technique during catheter access and dressing changes. Several guidelines help avoid complications:

- Use of antibiotic impregnated catheters
- Avoid use of femoral access sites
- Confirm patient allergies
- Review lab work for increased white blood cell count or blood glucose
- Closely monitor EKG, BP, temperature, and hemodynamics
- Frequently assess for chest pain, shortness of breath, and cyanosis
- Assess site every 4 hours and PRN for:
  - Erythema
  - Blanching
  - Breakdown
  - Drainage
  - Tenderness
  - Edema
  - Ecchymosis
  - Cording of a peripheral vein
- Investigate a patient who complains of:
  - Numbness, tingling
  - "Pins and needles"
  - Burning at site or along peripheral vein path
  - Headache or backache
- Minimize line access
- Change dressing per facility protocol and PRN
- Scrub port hub with chlorhexidine, or alcohol prep, for 15 seconds, allowing it to dry prior to access

- Flush all catheters and change caps per facility policy
- When changing tubing, place patient in Trendelenburg position

(Adapted from Alexander, 2006; Hadaway, 2007; Lee, 2009; Nettina, 2010.)

- Do not infuse solutions/medications with an osmolarity >600 mOsm/L through a PIV
- Do not infuse solutions/medications with a pH <5 or >9 via a PIV
- Immediately stop infusions/injections if patient complains of pain/burning
- Stop injection/infusion if infiltration is suspected

═══════════════════════════════*FAST FACTS in a NUTSHELL*

Following are examples of possible complications arising from IV therapy:

- Irregular heartbeat
- Infiltration
- Thrombophlebitis
- Hemorrhage
- Air embolus
- Hemo/pneumothorax
- Brachial plexus injury
- Extravasation
- Infection
- Thrombosis
- Volume overload
- Catheter migration, tear, or dislodgement
- Cardiac tamponade
- "Clotting" of line

Treatment of complications varies with the type encountered. For example, a declotting process can be initiated, with a physician order, which involves an alteplase instillation into the catheter. Pharmacy instructions must be strictly followed and all the alteplase must be aspirated from the line.

Treatment with phentolamine (Regitine) or hyaluronidase (Vitrase) can be performed for the infiltration and extravasation of certain drugs. For suspected catheter-related bloodstream infections, the IV access will be removed, the tip cultured, blood cultures drawn, and antibiotics administered.

IV MEDICATION ADMINISTRATION GUIDELINES

Administering IV medication safely requires knowledge, vigilance, and experience. Several implementations are suggested:

- Observe the five "rights" of medication administration: right drug, right patient, right dose, right time, and right route.
- Confirm patient allergies.
- Be knowledgeable about medications and solutions suspected to cause extravasation, such as:
  - Calcium chloride
  - Chemotherapy drugs
  - Diazepam
  - Dopamine
  - Gentamicin
  - Penicillin
  - Potassium chloride
  - Sodium bicarbonate
  - Vancomycin
  - Calcium gluconate
  - Dextrose
  - Dobutamine
  - Fat emulsion
  - Norepinephrine
  - Phenytoin
  - Propofol
  - TPN
  - Vasopressin
- Call pharmacy for questions/concerns regarding medications.
- Before administering each medication, assess IV access site for edema, vein cording, pain, discomfort, and drainage.
- Dilute medications, per manufacturer recommendation, with compatible IV solution.
- Examples of drugs that must be diluted prior to administration:
  - Hydrocortisone sodium succinate
  - Lorazepam
  - Morphine
  - Promethazine
  - Levothyroxine
  - Meperidine
  - Phenobarbital
- Educate patient and family regarding signs/symptoms of infiltration.

- Access IV using aseptic technique, being careful not to contaminate site.
- Clear air from tubing lines prior to connecting infusion to patient.
- Secure all IV connections.
- Use filters for solutions, if applicable.
- Check for positive blood return prior to IV medication administration.
- Immediately stop infusion/injection if pain, redness, or infiltration is noted.
- Notify physician of complications with IV access.
- Change IV bag every 24 hours.
- Change IV tubing and filter, if applicable, every 72 hours.
- During and after medication administration, monitor the patient for:
  - Anaphylaxis
  - EKG changes
  - Nausea/vomiting
  - Respiratory difficulties
  - Seizures
  - Rash/hives

(Adapted from Alexander, 2007; Chohan & Munden, 2007; Ehlers, 2007; Hadaway, 2007; Hodgson & Kizior, 2010; Lee, 2009; Nettina, 2010; Stillwell, 2006; Wyckoff et al., 2009.)

PATIENT CONTROLLED ANALGESIA

A patient who is alert, oriented, has manual dexterity, and can follow detailed instructions may be administered **patient controlled analgesia (PCA), a short-term option for pain management.** PCA is a great modality for treating post-operative pain when the patient is able to actively participate and is monitored properly. However, several errors can occur with this treatment, necessitating familiarity with its use, pump programming, required patient monitoring, and proper documentation.

PCA is administered through an IV access, usually a PIV. Infusion via an epidural is also possible. A computerized pump and the patient control analgesia, allowing active participation in care. The patient operates a button that is depressed when medication is desired. **The drugs routinely utilized are morphine, hydromorphone (Dilaudid), and fentanyl (Sublimaze).**

Orders are received from a physician, frequently an anesthesiologist, and programmed into the pump by an RN. **Orders include the medication, its concentration, a loading dose, bolus (demand) dose, dose interval, and lock-out interval,** which is how much of the drug the patient can receive in 1 hour, regardless of how many times the demand button is depressed. Basal rates are no longer given.

FAST FACTS in a NUTSHELL

Per Joint Commission recommendations, a pre-filled syringe or bag is sent from the pharmacy with a standard concentration of the medication ordered. The key needed to access the pump is often kept in an automated mediation dispensing system or with the charge nurse.

When filling and programming a PCA pump, a second RN must verify the order and the programming. Two nurses must also verify a change in settings and confirm programming upon unit transfer and at shift change.

Once the orders and programming are confirmed, **education is provided to the patient and family regarding PCA use.** It is imperative that no one except the patient pushes the demand button, even when the patient is asleep. Family members with good intentions might want to do this; however, they should be informed of the potentional complications caused by overmedication.

Continuous monitoring of patients receiving PCA is vital. Pulse oximetry and/or capnography can be used to monitor ventilations, along with a nursing evaluation of respiratory status. Blood pressure, heart rate, and pain should also be frequently assessed. Implementation of a sedation tool, such as the Richmond Agitation Sedation Scale, is required and should be documented every 2–4 hours or per facility policy.

When a change in patient status is observed, the physician should be notified. If warranted, the infusion will be changed or stopped. Familiarity with sedation reversal drugs, such as naloxone (Narcan), is essential.

PCA administration has other side effects, in addition to respiratory depression and sedation, related to the drugs used. Constipation, nausea, vomiting, and itching are often experienced. Medications and treatments can be administered to combat these issues.

Critical Care Equipment
Competencies

10

The Respiratory Station

INTRODUCTION

Patients in the critical care unit suffer from a multitude of illnesses that involve the respiratory system. Even if the underlying pathology is not of a respiratory nature, lung function and breathing mechanisms are often affected. Prevalent disorders, such as congestive heart failure, acute respiratory distress syndrome, pulmonary edema, chronic obstructive pulmonary disease, and asthma, wreak havoc on the entire body.

When exacerbations of such ailments compromise a patient's ability to sustain adequate oxygenation, supplementation and assistance are required. These can occur in several ways, ranging from the application of a simple nasal cannula to endotracheal intubation and the use of a ventilator. Many factors dictate which type of treatment the patient receives.

In this chapter, you will learn:

1. The avenues used to provide oxygenation.
2. Techniques to assist with intubation and extubation.
3. How to care for endotracheal and tracheostomy tubes.
4. The basics of mechanical ventilation and related complication management.

113

SUPPLEMENTAL OXYGENATION

When a patient is suffering from a condition that causes an inability to get rid of carbon dioxide (CO_2) or problems getting enough oxygen (O_2) into their system, supplemental oxygenation and medical treatment are required. **O_2 is administered via a delivery device, with levels ranging from 24% to 100%.** The equipment frequently used to provide O_2 includes a nasal cannula, facemask, and nasotracheal or orotracheal tube. These may be connected directly to O_2 via tubing or attached to various machines, such as a non-invasive positive pressure ventilation device or a mechanical ventilator. **The type of O_2 supplementation is determined by several parameters,** including saturation of oxyhemoglobin (SpO_2), arterial blood gases (ABGs), respirations per minute, use of accessory muscles for breathing, cyanosis, mental status, vital signs, hemodynamics, and the physician's clinical judgment.

O_2 delivery is initiated via the least-invasive option that provides adequate treatment. **The patient is also treated medically to correct the underlying cause of the respiratory dysfunction.** Frequent assessments are performed. Based on the findings, O_2 and medical modalities are adjusted to accommodate progress or deterioration.

INTUBATION

Endotracheal Tube

When noninvasive techniques such as nasal cannulas, facemasks, continuous positive airway pressure (CPAP), and/or biphasic positive airway pressure (BiPAP) fail to improve a patient's condition or the initial assessment warrants, intubation is performed via the nasal or oral route.

The oral route is preferred, unless contraindicated, because of reduced risk of bleeding and sinusitis, along with easier insertion. Intubation allows for maintenance of a patent airway, deep suctioning and improved secretion removal, and lower aspiration risk.

================================*FAST FACTS in a NUTSHELL*

Some general parameters indicating that intubation is required include:

- PaO_2 < 50 mmHg with FiO_2 > 60
- PaO_2 > 50 mmHg but pH < 7.25
- Respiratory rate (RR) > 35 breaths per minute
- Vital capacity < 2 × tidal volume (VT)

In most states, **intubation is not within the scope of practice for an RN**. However, nurses frequently assist with the procedure. Proper preparation improves the ease of artificial airway insertion. The equipment needed for intubation is:

- Resuscitation bag with mask
- Laryngoscope with functioning light; curved blade (Macintosh) and straight blade (Miller)
- Cuffed endotracheal tubes (ETTs) in a variety of sizes: 6.0, 7.0, 8.0, and 9.0 mm
- ETT stylet
- Oral airway, in a variety of sizes
- Tape or facility-approved ETT stabilizer set
- Sterile lubricant
- 10-cc syringe
- Suction set-up: functioning suction source, canister, tubing, tonsil suction, sterile suction catheters, sterile gloves, sterile saline
- Sterile towels
- Gloves
- Masks and eye protection, or face shield
- CO_2 detector
- Stethoscope
- Procedural medications, if ordered

================================= *FAST FACTS in a NUTSHELL*

The following pre-procedural patient preparation for intubation should be completed:

- Confirm identity via two patient identifiers.
- Confirm informed consent, unless an emergency condition exists.
- Provide patient and family with education, if possible.
- Remove bridges, partials, or dentures. Store and label properly.

When the practitioner arrives, assist as needed. Assistance can include:

- Removing the headboard from the bed
- Assembling laryngoscope and blade
- Checking the cuff of the requested ETT for leaks by inflating the bulb with 5–10 cc of air via the 10-cc syringe, while maintaining ETT sterility
- Inserting the stylet into the selected ETT, ensuring that the tip of the stylet does not protrude from the tip of the ETT
- Completing a "time-out"
- Pre-medicating the patient, as ordered, with sedatives, anxiolytics, narcotics, and/or paralytics
- Placing the patient in the "sniffing" position, if no cervical injury is noted
- Performing jaw thrust, if a cervical injury is suspected
- Oxygenating the patient via the resuscitation bag and mask with 100% O_2
- Applying external cricoid pressure
- Once intubation is achieved, attaching the resuscitation bag to the ETT, ensuring no inward or outward movement
- Inflating the cuff with 5–10 cc of air, post-ETT insertion as directed

- Inserting an oral airway (bite block), if required
- Observing for chest rise
- Auscultating lung fields and epigastric area
- Applying and checking CO_2 detector. In most facilities, the cap will be purple, then turn gold/yellow when exposed to CO_2
- Noting the distance from the tip of the ETT to the lips
- Securing the ETT with tape or facility-approved stabilizer
- Confirming that a chest x-ray has been ordered and/or performed
- Attaching ventilator tubing
- Confirming ventilator settings with practitioner

(Adapted from Alspach, 2006; Ehlers, 2007; Foreman et al., 2010; Nettina, 2010; Stillwell, 2006; Wyckoff et al., 2009.)

After the tube has been secured and placement verified, **document the type and size of the ETT, location at lips, cuff pressure, and tolerance.**

═══════════════════════*FAST FACTS in a NUTSHELL*

Complications associated with endotracheal intubation include right mainstem intubation, greater mucous production, aspiration, atelectasis, pneumonia, vocal cord ulceration, laryngospasm/edema/stenosis, tracheal ischemia/necrosis/stenosis/dilation, tracheoesophageal fistula, and innominate artery erosion.

ETT Maintenance and Suctioning

After intubation, **ETT maintenance and suctioning are required.** Keys to maintaining an ETT are the following:

- Auscultate lung fields and assess respiratory status frequently.

- Notify the physician if absent breath sounds are noted; anticipate chest x-ray and tube repositioning.
- Assess tube placement and position at lips.
- Assess oral mucosa.
- Reposition the ETT from one side of mouth to the other to prevent pressure ulcers of mouth/lips, at facility-approved intervals.
- Perform oral care 2 times per day and as needed.
- Moisturize lips frequently.
- Suction mouth/pharynx as needed.
- Monitor tube cuff pressure; a manometer may be used.
- Ensure adequate O_2 humidification.
- Change patient position every 2 hours, unless contraindicated.
- Document assessment findings, care completed, patient tolerance, changes, etc.

Suctioning is performed to remove secretions. This is a sterile procedure completed via a single-use, or a closed-suction catheter system. Several steps are followed when performing single-use ETT suctioning alone, as detailed in Figure 10.1. If another staff member is available to assist, suctioning is a bit simpler to complete, and sterility is easily maintained. Follow manufacturer and facility guidelines when using a closed-suction catheter system.

Coughing can be expected during suctioning. However, **if the patient develops intolerance to the procedure, stop.** Assess the situation and provide care as needed. Suctioning has potential for complications, such as arrhythmias, bronchospasm or laryngospasm, hypertension, hypotension, hypoxemia, and increased intracranial pressure (ICP).

Tracheal Tubes

When intubation via the nasal or oral route is contraindicated or impossible, or a patient requires long-term intubation, **a percutaneous tracheal tube can be inserted.**

Figure 10.1 Steps for Performing Single-Use Catheter ETT Suctioning

1. Gather supplies:
   a. No. 14 or No. 16 sterile suction catheters (normal adult)
   b. Sterile gloves
   c. Sterile towel
   d. Suction source
   e. Sterile water
   f. Resuscitation bag connected to 100% O_2
   g. Sterile cup
   h. Sterile water-soluble lubricant
   i. PPE
2. Perform hand hygiene and don appropriate PPE.
3. Provide patient education.
4. Closely monitor vital signs, SpO_2, hemodynamics, etc. throughout and following suction procedure.
5. Turn on suction and set vacuum to 80–120 mmHg.
6. Attach the connecting tubing to the suction vacuum, and put the other end in an easy place to locate.
7. Maintain aseptic technique at all times.
8. Put the patient in semi- or high-Fowler's position, unless contraindicated.
9. Open sterile towel; place on patient's chest.
10. Open suction catheter on a clean table; use the inside wrapper as a sterile field.
11. Squeeze water-soluble lubricant onto sterile field, avoiding outer edge.
12. Set up sterile cup, open sterile water, and fill cup.

Continued

Figure 10.1 *Continued*

13. Put on sterile gloves. Maintain dominant hand as sterile, nondominant hand as nonsterile.
14. With sterile hand, remove suction catheter from package and curl around fingers.
15. With nonsterile hand, connect suction tubing to suction catheter.
16. With nonsterile hand, disconnect patient from O_2 source and hyperoxygenate with resuscitation bag and 100% O_2 for 30 seconds.
17. Remove resuscitation bag.
18. Using sterile hand, dip catheter in sterile lubricant, applying a small amount.
19. Easily insert suction catheter into the ETT, without applying suction, until slight resistance is met.
20. Pull back 1 cm.
21. While withdrawing the catheter, apply either continuous or intermittent suction. Rotate the catheter while suctioning. Complete this pass in 10 seconds or less.
22. Hyperoxygenate patient for 30 seconds.
23. Clean suction catheter between passes by inserting tip into sterile water and suctioning up a small amount.
24. If needed, suction patient again, following steps 16 to 21.
25. Stop suctioning when no secretions remain, four passes have been completed, or patient shows signs of procedure intolerance.
26. Hyperoxygenate patient.
27. Return patient to ventilator or other oxygen-delivery device.
28. Suction oropharynx and oral cavity.

Continued

Figure 10.1   *Continued*

29. Auscultate lung fields.
30. Reposition patient, if needed.
31. Document procedure, sputum/secretion app-
    earance, and patient tolerance.

Note: Refer to facility policy/procedure for specific/additional guidelines.

(Adapted from Alspach, 2006; Ehlers, 2007; Nettina, 2010, Stillwell, 2006.)

This procedure is usually performed in the operating room, but, in rare situations, may occur elsewhere in the hospital.

Tracheal tubes are shorter than ETTs, may be cuffed or uncuffed and fenestrated or nonfenestrated. Some have an inner cannula and/or contain valves. Most can be downsized, as tolerated. Common sizes are 5.0, 6.0, 7.0, and 8.0 mm. The tube is secured via ties, tapes, and/or a facility-approved securing device.

Tracheal tube care and maintenance are very similar to those of an ETT. Some guidelines of importance include the following:

- Measure cuff pressure every 8 to 12 hours and as needed. Recommended pressure is about 18 mmHg, unless otherwise ordered. Do not exceed 25 mmHg.
- A manometer may be used.
- Assess stoma with care. Keep it clean and dry.
- Use aseptic technique during stoma and outer cannula care.
- Do not use powder or oil-based creams/lotions near stoma.
- Inner cannula may be disposable or reusable.
- If reusable, the inner cannula should be cleaned per facility protocol and as needed.

- When changing a disposable inner cannula, touch only the outer locking portion; the inner portion is considered sterile.
- Do not change a single cannula tube or outer cannula of double-cannula tube; the doctor usually does this.
- Keep extra inner cannulas at bedside.
- Keep an extra tracheostomy tube of the same size and type at the bedside.
- Keep tube obturator at the bedside.
- Check ties/securing device often.
- When changing tracheostomy ties or securing device, try to have another staff member at the bedside to assist.
- When changing ties or securing device alone, attach new ties/device before removing old ones.

(Adapted from Alspach, 2006; Ehlers, 2007; Nettina, 2010; Tracheostomy Care Handbook, 1998; Stillwell, 2006.)

Suctioning a trach tube is similar to suctioning an ETT. Check facility procedure guidelines and manufacturer recommendations for proper suction catheter size.

═══════════════════════════*FAST FACTS in a NUTSHELL*

Possible complications related to a tracheostomy include hemorrhage, stoma infection, tracheitis, pneumonia, subglottic edema, mediastinal emphysema, pneumothorax, tracheal stenosis/necrosis/dilation, larynx stenosis, tracheoesophageal fistula, vocal cord ulceration, innominate artery erosion, and damage to neck structures in close proximity to the stoma.

Patients who are intubated, or trached, have limited communication. The health care team is responsible for providing emotional support and education to the patient and family. A means of communication should be developed, such as hand signals, head nodding, blinks, and/or a communication board. The call bell should remain within reach.

MECHANICAL VENTILATION

Mechanical ventilators are common in the ICU. There are two major categories: negative external pressure and positive pressure. The latter is most frequently used. Its mechanism applies positive pressure to airways in a programmed pattern. Oxygen is pushed into the lungs, causing alveolar expansion. An artificial airway is usually needed. The physician adjusts trigger, gas delivery, and cycling to attain desired outcomes.

A negative external pressure ventilator functions to imitate spontaneous breathing. Sometimes referred to as an iron lung, this vent encompasses the whole body, except the head and neck. A few variations exist, all requiring a tight seal around the chest. No artificial airway is required. These machines are not usually found in the nursing unit, as they treat specific issues, such as neuromuscular diseases.

There are four types of positive pressure vents: pressure-, volume-, time-, and flow-cycled. A pressure-cycled machine presses air into the lungs until a set airway pressure has been met. A volume-cycled mechanism delivers air until a programmed volume has been met, allowing VT to remain unchanged. Time-cycled vents force air into the lungs for a certain amount of time, with the VT and pressure adjusted for each patient. Flow-cycled machines deliver air to the lungs, during inspiration, until a specific flow is met.

The ways to control a ventilator vary with the type of mechanism and its selected mode. Some examples of ventilator modes include the following:

- *Continuous mandatory ventilation (CMV):* Respirations are provided at a set VT and RR. Spontaneous breaths are blocked. Patients receiving this type of mechanical ventilation are usually sedated and often given paralytics. It is not a commonly used method.

- *Assist-controlled ventilation (A/C):* Allows the patient to initiate breaths. O_2 is provided at a set VT and a specific number of respirations are machine provided. The pressure is variable. Patient-initiated breaths receive the same VT as machine-provided breaths.
- *Intermittent mandatory ventilation (IMV):* Allows spontaneous respirations. Programmed volume, pressure, and number of breaths are also delivered.
- *Synchronized IMV (SIMV):* A type of IMV. Machine-provided breaths are synchronized with spontaneous breaths. Patient-initiated breaths receive patient-controlled VT.
- *Pressure support ventilation (PSV):* The patient must initiate every breath. The vent provides positive pressure. VT and RR are patient controlled, and often used with SIMV or weaning.
- *Continuous positive airway pressure (CPAP):* Positive pressure is exerted and continued during spontaneous breathing; it is frequently used for weaning and contraindicated in ICP.
- *Pressure-controlled/inverse-ratio ventilation (PC/IRV):* Spontaneous breathing is blocked. Pressure and RR are machine controlled. Longer inspiratory versus expiratory time provides greater ventilation distribution. Patients receive sedation and paralytics.

(Adapted from Alspach, 2006; Nettina, 2010; Stillwell, 2006; Wyckoff et al., 2009.)

Ventilator settings, such as VT, I/R ratio, oxygen concentration (FiO_2), and positive end-expiratory pressure (PEEP), are adjusted to achieve desired outcomes. Humidification is used for all patients. **The combination of mode, function, and setting is determined by physician** preference, expertise, the disease or condition, and available treatment modalities.

Some common ventilator settings are defined and detailed below:

- *FiO$_2$*: Generally set to keep PaO$_2$ > 55 mmHg and SaO$_2$ > 88%, with a maximum of 0.5 to 0.65. The lowest amount required should be used to prevent O$_2$ toxicity.
- *RR*: Usually 8 to 20 breaths per minute.
- *PEEP*: The amount of positive pressure applied by the vent at end expiration. It affects functional residual capacity and compliance, and may reduce the amount of FiO$_2$ needed. Often set between 3 and 20 cm of H$_2$O, with the lowest amount necessary used to prevent barotrauma.
- *Flow rate:* Usually 40–100 L/min. It is the inspiratory volume that is delivered in a pre-set amount of time to allow for appropriate exhalation.
- *VT:* Usually 6–12 ml/kg. It is the amount of gas provided with each respiration.
- *Pressure support (PS)*: Positive pressure "assistance" provided by the vent on inspiration to decrease the amount of work required of the patient.
- *I/E ratio*: 1:2, 1:3.
- *Sensitivity*: Usually −0.50 to −1.5 cm H$_2$O. It is the level at which the vent senses the patient initiating a breath and provides support.

(Adapted from Alspach, 2006; Ehlers, 2007; Nettina, 2010; Stillwell, 2006; Wyckoff et al., 2009.)

A ventilator can take measurements directly from the patient. Minute volume (MV; which is usually 6–10 L/min and defined as the amount air inhaled or exhaled by the patient), RR, and VT are examples. The machine can also determine plateau pressure, an estimate of alveolar pressure at end expiration with a goal of 30–35 cm of H$_2$O.

The effectiveness of mechanical ventilation is evaluated in several ways. Physical assessment, ABG interpretation (discussed in Chapter 11), hemodynamics, lab results (e.g., hematology and electrolytes), pulmonary function tests, and assessment of sputum are all keys to understanding ventilatory success.

=== *FAST FACTS in a NUTSHELL*

Several items and activities are involved in caring for a patient requiring mechanical ventilation. Some equipment to have at the bedside includes a resuscitation bag, suction equipment, PPE, and a stethoscope.

Monitoring a vented patient involves great diligence and documentation. Measurements, observations, outcomes, and settings to record include:

- ABG results, including source (e.g., radial artery)
- Vent settings: mode, VT, temperature, RR, FiO_2, peak inflation limit, PEEP, alarm status, and I/E ratio
- Patient: PEEP, MV, RR, and compliance
- Pulse oximetry (SpO_2)
- End-tidal CO_2, ($PetCO_2$)
- Hemodynamics
- Patient comfort

=== *FAST FACTS in a NUTSHELL*

Many complications and side effects are related to mechanical ventilation. The most well known is ventilator-associated pneumonia (VAP). Others include:

- Decreased cardiac output
- Pneumothorax
- Atelectasis
- Tracheoesophageal fistula
- Inability to wean from vent
- Respiratory alkalosis
- Gastric ulcer/bleeding
- Agitation
- Dysrhythmias
- Subcutaneous emphysema
- Tracheal damage
- O_2 toxicity
- Respiratory acidosis
- Fluid retention
- Ileus
- Deep vein thrombosis

Complications related to mechanical ventilation are treated according to the symptoms presented. It is important to notify the physician of acute changes in assessment, ABGs, lab results, ventilatory status, and so on. Guidelines for side-effect and complication management include the following:

- For decreased cardiac output: use a modified Trendelenburg position, provide intravenous (IV) fluids to improve preload, and titrate PEEP carefully.
- Barotrauma prevention: Use the lowest PEEP level possible.
- Atelectasis prevention: Use low VT, ensure proper humidification, perform tracheal suction as needed; perform chest physical therapy and frequent patient repositioning.
- Tracheal damage prevention: Closely monitor ETT/ trach cuff pressure; avoid pulling and excess handling of the ETT.
- O_2 toxicity prevention: monitor ABGs (see Chapter 11); use lowest FiO_2 possible.
- Improve the ability to wean from vent with proper nutritional support.
- Respiratory acidosis treatment: Treat underlying cause.
- Respiratory alkalosis treatment: Lower RR and VT; add mechanical dead space.
- Gastrointestinal issues: Administer antacids and histamine antagonists; perform hemoccult/gastroccult, test pH of stomach contents.

(Adapted from Alspach, 2006; Ehlers, 2007; Nettina, 2010; Tracheostomy Care Handbook, 1998; Stillwell, 2006; Wyckoff et al., 2009.)

Prevention of VAP involves a multilayered approach, involving several interventions:

- Maintaining aseptic technique during ETT/trach suctioning, avoiding use of saline lavage, if possible.

- Frequent and complete oral care.
- Chest physical therapy.
- Practicing proper isolation precautions.
- Routine cultures of patients and ventilators.
- Appropriate antibiotic administration, if applicable.
- Close monitoring of lab work pertaining to infection.
- Awareness of assessment indications of infection.
- Limited contact between patient and staff/visitors.
- Changing of reservoir water per facility policy.
- Emptying of the water collected in the vent tubing, because of condensation, every 2 hours and as needed. Drain the water into a collection cup and empty. **Do not** drain the water into humidifier.

(Adapted from Alspach, 2006; Centers for Disease Control and Prevention, 2003; Ehlers, 2007; Martin, 2010; Nettina, 2010; Pear, 2007; Stillwell, 2006.)

FAST FACTS in a NUTSHELL

Patients sometimes suffer from agitation and fight or "buck" the vent. Provide comfort with proper management and interventions:

- Assess the patient and ventilator, noting any changes.
- Provide reassurance and education to the patient.
- Assess ABGs.
- Suction the ETT/trach and check the cuff.
- Provide 100% O_2 via resuscitation bag or ventilator.
- Adjust vent settings as needed.
- Administer sedation, if indicated, following adequate evaluation of situation.

Ventilators have alarms that frequently go off. The following are common alarms and their corresponding causes:

- High RR: Pain/anxiety, fever, hypoxia, buildup of secretions.

- Apnea: No spontaneous respirations noted by machine during a programmed time limit. Immediately assess the patient.
- Low exhaled volume: Loose/disconnected vent tubing, leak in ETT/trach cuff, leak in chest tube, electrical supply problem with vent, or malfunctioning vent.
- Low inspiratory pressure: Loose/disconnected vent tubing, increased spontaneous breathing, displaced ETT/trach, vent malfunction, leak in vent tubing.
- High pressure: The most frequent alarm. Possible causes include right mainstem intubation, kinked vent/airway tubing, patient biting the ETT, cough, buildup of secretions, bronchospasm, pneumothorax, lowered lung compliance, condensation build-up in tubing.
- Thermometer alert: Assess the in-line thermometer.

Whenever an alarm, or complication, is encountered with the ventilator, **assess the patient first.** If needed, provide manual respirations via the resuscitation bag. This supports the patient with adequate oxygenation during troubleshooting. **Consult with respiratory therapists often.** Supplemental oxygenation is their area of expertise, and it is very helpful to have their additional knowledge at the bedside.

EXTUBATION

Extubation is the ultimate goal for a patient undergoing mechanical ventilation. Many clinicians refer to extubation as liberation or weaning. The steps that are followed to achieve this goal should be completed in order; however, setbacks, comorbidities, and changes in underlying conditions call for the steps to shift. Often, ICU patients make multiple attempts before freedom from the ventilator and ETT/trach is complete.

The type of weaning trial is determined by the ventilator settings the patient has previously tolerated and the physician's orders. A T-piece (a T-shaped airway adapter attached to high-humidity O_2), CPAP, IMV, or SIMV are all types of weaning. Pressure support may be added to IMV or SIMV trials. A respiratory therapist will assist with ventilator weaning protocols. **The weaning process may take as little as an hour to several days, according to policy and patient tolerance.** It should be initiated when the patient is well rested.

Before instituting a weaning trial, confirm that the patient has received medications that may improve tolerance and lung function, such as albuterol (AccuNeb, Proventil HFA), beclomethasone (Beconase AQ, Qvar), cromolyn (Nasalcrom, Intal), fluticasone (Flonase, Veramyst), formoterol (Foradil Aerolizer, Perforomist), hydrocortisone (Solu-Cortef, Cortef), ipratropium (Atrovent), methylprednisolone (Solu-Medrol), montelukast (Singulair), prednisone (Sterapred), salmeterol (Serevent Diskus), terbutaline (Brethine), theophylline (Theo-24, Theolair), or tiotropium (Spiriva). These medications are administered in various ways: via inhalation, IV push, orally, subcutaneously, or nasal spray, depending on the drug and treatment type ordered.

Certain parameters should be met before attempting to wean a patient from a mechanical ventilator:

- The underlying disease (the reason for the need for a vent) is resolved.
- Respiratory system strength and nutritional status are sufficient.
- PEEP is ≤5 cm H_2O.
- FiO_2 is ≤50%.
- PaO_2 is at least 55–60 mmHg.
- Hemodynamics and vital signs are stable.
- ABGs and hemoglobin are within normal limits.
- Patient is awake, alert, and compliant.
- Ventilatory measurements are within an acceptable range:
  - MV <10.
  - Max. inspiratory pressure is below –20 cm H_2O.
  - Spontaneous VT >5 ml/kg.

- Spontaneous RR ranges between 12 and 30.
- Vital capacity >10 ml/kg body weight.
- Positive expiratory pressure >+30 cm H_2O.

The primary steps in ventilator weaning are as follows:

1. Confirm physician's order and verify identity via two patient identifiers.
2. Educate the patient/family.
3. Position patient upright.
4. Document current vital signs and hemodynamics.
5. Have resuscitation bag available.
6. Measure MV, RR, VT, maximum inspiratory pressure, VC, and maximum ventilatory pressure from patient-initiated breaths.
7. Initiate physician-specified weaning trial settings.
8. Return to baseline vent settings for:
   a. VT < 250–300 ml in an adult patient
   b. RR increase >10 breaths per minute or RR >30
   c. Increasing $PaCO_2$
   d. Decreasing pH
   e. Lowered SpO_2
   f. Increase in ratio of inspiratory time to total duration of respiration
   g. Anxiety, sweating, or fatigue
   h. Change in level of consciousness
   i. EKG changes
   j. Blood pressure change of 20 mmHg systolic or 10 mmHg diastolic
   k. Heart rate change of 20 beats/min or heart rate >110
   l. Acute change in hemodynamics
   m. Abnormal chest-wall motion
9. Repeat ABGs at ordered intervals.
10. Continue monitoring the patient.

(Adapted from Alspach, 2006; Ehlers, 2007; Nettina, 2010; Stillwell, 2006; Wyckoff et al., 2009.)

Once weaning trials have proven successful, either a physician or respiratory therapist will extubate the patient. A 10-cc syringe (to deflate the cuff), suction, a resuscitation bag, appropriate PPE, and intended O_2 delivery device, such as a facemask or nasal cannula, should be at the bedside. When extubation is complete, the patient must be closely monitored to ensure adequate tolerance and ventilation.

11

Arterial Blood Gases, Arterial Lines, and Pulmonary Artery Catheters

INTRODUCTION

Many types of equipment are used in the intensive care unit (ICU). Surgeries, procedures, nursing interventions, medication administration, and medical treatments are performed in an effort to improve the patient's condition. Some of these are based on test results and the assessment of hemodynamic values.

An arterial blood gas (ABG), obtained from an arterial line, is used to assess oxygen exchange and acid–base balance. Intubation, extubation, and ventilator settings are generally determined after the evaluation of an ABG.

Arterial lines and pulmonary artery (PA) catheters provide valuable information to the health care team regarding the patient's respiratory, hydration, and hemodynamic status. These invasive catheters are inserted by an advanced practitioner, using sterile technique, and are found in just about every ICU.

In this chapter you will learn:

1. The ABCs of ABGs.
2. The ins and outs of arterial lines and PA catheters.

ARTERIAL BLOOD GASES

An ABG sample is commonly used to evaluate ventilation and acid–base balance. The parameters measured for an ABG are pH, bicarbonate (HCO_3), partial pressure of oxygen (PO_2), arterial oxygen saturation (SaO_2), partial pressure of carbon dioxide (PCO_2), and base excess (BE).

═══════════════════════════════*FAST FACTS in a NUTSHELL*

Normal Blood Gas Ranges for an Adult

pH: 7.35–7.45
PO_2: 80–100 mmHg
SaO_2: >95%
PCO_2: 35–45 mmHg
HCO_3: 22–26 mEq/L
BE: –2 to +2

Note: These are the arterial ranges at sea level.

ABGs are obtained from an arterial stick or an access device, referred to as a vamp, which allows blood to be drawn from an arterial line (A-line). For patients who require frequent ABG analysis, insertion of an arterial line is performed to reduce the number of sticks a patient receives.

It is within the registered nurse's scope of practice to perform an arterial puncture when specifically trained. However, in most facilities, a physician or respiratory therapist performs this procedure. For detailed instructions on performing an arterial stick, ask the hospital's nursing education department or refer to the *Lippincott Manual of Nursing Practice*. Before performing this procedure, confirm facility policy guidelines.

Patient education, preparation for an arterial puncture, and A-line insertion are frequently performed by the ICU nurse. Aseptic technique is used during this process, and appropriate PPE (see Chapter 8) is needed. **The Allen** test should be completed before any type of radial artery access.

Protocols for Performing an ABG Blood Draw From Either an Arterial Stick or an A-Line

- A heparinized blood gas syringe is required.
- Note facility policy to ensure the proper amount of blood to be wasted prior to the specimen draw.
- Remove all air from the syringe.
- Place the specimen on ice immediately after it is drawn.
- Document the time and date of the specimen, patient's temperature, type of O_2 delivery device, O_2 amount, and vent settings, if applicable.
- Wait 20 minutes before obtaining blood for ABG analysis following any type of O_2 change. This ensures adequate time for changes to be reflected.

Following an arterial stick, pressure is applied to the site until hemostasis, approximately 5 minutes. If anticoagulants have been administered, expect the time to increase to 10 to 15 minutes. A secure, noncircumferential dressing is applied to the site once hemostasis is achieved. A pressure dressing is not applied. **Monitor the site** for a palpable pulse, bleeding, ecchymosis, changes in skin color, coolness of the extremity, and patient complaints of numbness or tingling.

A-LINE

If the patient is to have an A-line inserted, a small-bore flex-ible-tip catheter is placed in the radial, femoral, brachial, or axillary artery. **The radial is most desirable for infection prevention purposes.** When preparing to assist with an **A-line insertion, note that it is a sterile procedure.**

A few sutures are made at the insertion site to help keep the catheter in place. An occlusive dressing covers the site. The catheter is connected to specific tubing and a facility-specified heparinized saline. A pressure bag is applied to the outside of the bag, applying 300 mmHg of force on the fluid, maintaining a flush of approximately 3 cc/hour to ensure line patency.

A single transducer system is attached to the line to monitor blood pressure (BP). A "box" attached to the monitor, a transducer cable, the transducer, and an air-fluid interface (stop-cock) are parts of the system. A stop-cock holder is often used via an IV pole. The transducer system is calibrated prior to A-line insertion per manufacturer/facility instructions.

The **stop-cock should be level with the phlebostatic axis to zero the monitoring system after the A-line is inserted.** The phlebostatic axis is approximately the level of the right atrium (RA). It can be located by finding the fourth intercostal space, midaxillary line. Once zeroed, the square-wave test will be completed:

1. Initiate the fast flush mechanism.
2. Flush rapidly for 1/2 a second.
3. Note the square-wave pattern on monitor. The waveform should rise quickly, level out (become flat) on top, then drop back down, looking like a square box on the A-line tracing (Figure 11.1).
4. Next, observe for an adequate A-line waveform.

(Adapted from Ehlers, 2007; Mobile Infirmary Medical Center, n.d.; Stillwell, 2006.)

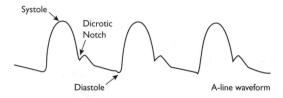

FIGURE 11.1   A-line waveform.

Ensure that A-line alarms are on and set to appropriate parameters for the patient. Re-level the transducer with patient/transducer movement and PRN. Check stopcocks/connections frequently to ensure secureness. Dressings are changed according to the type of dressing applied and facility policy.

A-line waveforms may become "damp," which means that it appears either too short or too tall. Steps can be taken to correct these readings:

1. Assess the patient.
2. Perform non-invasive BP (NIBP) reading.
3. *Overdamped waveform:* A short, peaked waveform with minimal dicrotic notch. This depicts a low systolic BP with a high diastolic BP in relation to a true reading.
   a. Assess pressure bag for 300 mmHg pressure and adequate reserve in flush bag.
   b. Complete square-wave test.
   c. Check insertion site for catheter position, drainage, kinks, and so on.
   d. Assess tubing and A-line system for bubbles, and clear (do not flush air toward patient), if needed.
   e. Check system for leaks, disconnection, and so on.
   f. Aspirate blood from tubing (using aseptic technique), then flush the line well.
4. *Underdamped waveform:* A tall, peaked waveform. This depicts a high systolic BP with a low diastolic BP in relation to a true reading.
   a. Assess patient for low BP; check other hemodynamics if possible.
   b. Complete square-wave test.
   c. Assess system for air bubbles, and clear (do not flush air toward patient), if needed.
   d. Assess length of tubing and make shorter, if possible.
   e. Note number of stopcocks in use and decrease, if possible.

(Adapted from Alspach, 2006; Chohan & Munden, 2007; Ehlers, 2007; Kerner, 2007; Nettina, 2010; Stillwell, 2006.)

If problems persist, notify the physician. The catheter may need to be removed. **It is within the registered nurse's scope of practice to discontinue or remove an arterial line.** The procedure is as follows:

1. Confirm physician order.
2. Verify patient identity via two identifiers.
3. Review patient's coagulation and hematology results.
4. Provide patient and family education.
5. Put on necessary PPE.
6. Remove dressing.
7. Aspirate 3–5 ml of blood from the port into a syringe; leave syringe attached.
8. Apply pressure 1 to 2 finger widths above catheter insertion site.
9. Remove catheter in one swift stroke, noting if catheter tip is intact.
10. Apply pressure to site with a sterile 4 × 4.
11. Hold pressure until hemostasis; 5 to 10 minutes, or longer if needed.
12. Apply a transparent dressing to site. Do not wrap dressing circumferentially around the wrist. No pressure dressing is needed.
13. Limit patient activity with associated limb for approximately 1 hour.
14. Continue to monitor BP with an NIBP.

(Adapted from Alexander, 2006; Chohan & Munden, 2007; Ehlers, 2007; Kerner, 2007; Stillwell, 2006.)

Assess the site frequently for a palpable pulse, bleeding, ecchymosis, changes in skin color, coolness of the extremity, and patient complaints of numbness or tingling. Document education, procedure, and patient tolerance.

A vamp is often attached to an A-line. It makes maintaining aseptic technique easier and reduces the amount of blood wasted. If this type of device is not available, a port for blood draws can be used to access the line. Follow aseptic technique and ensure that an adequate flush follows blood withdrawal regardless of the method used. For systems without a vamp, apply a new, nonvented, sterile cap to the port with each access.

PULMONARY ARTERY CATHETER

A pulmonary artery (PA) catheter is used to obtain several hemodynamic measurements, such as PA pressure (PA), PA wedge pressure (PAWP), right atrial pressure (RAP), and cardiac output (CO). From these readings, other hemodynamics can be calculated, such as cardiac index (CI), stroke volume (SV), systemic venous resistance (SVR), and left ventricular stroke work index (LVSWI).

A PA catheter is placed into the right side of the heart via a large vein, such as the jugular, subclavian, or femoral, by a physician or advanced practitioner using aseptic technique. The right internal jugular is the most common insertion site because it is the shortest, straightest, large venous access to the heart. An introducer is inserted into the vein before the actual PA catheter.

The distal tip of this flow-directed, balloon-tipped catheter rests in the PA. The PA catheter is attached to a monitoring system that has been properly calibrated to allow for accurate readings. There may be as many as six lumens on the catheter, and a thermistor lumen is used for CO monitoring. Some have a pacing lumen and/or a mixed-venous oxygen saturation (SvO_2) measurement port. Several of the ports allow access for medication administration.

Normal saline bags, wrapped with pressure bags, provide a small, constant flush of fluid to the catheter tip to maintain patency. The saline is infused using semirigid tubing. Transducers are involved in PA catheter set-up and monitoring.

The PA catheter is used in many situations, such as acute myocardial infarction, burns, cardiovascular disease, heart failure, monitoring of vasoactive drug effectiveness, pulmonary issues, sepsis, shock, respiratory failure, valve disease, and whenever hemodynamic pressures are needed to assist with appropriate medical interventions.

Assisting with the insertion of a PA catheter at the bedside requires several steps:

1. Verify patient identity via two facility-approved identifiers. Confirm consent.
2. Provide patient/family education.
3. Zero and calibrate the bedside monitor and pressure monitoring system.
4. Apply a pressure bag to a facility-specified fluid for the monitoring system, and inflate to 300 mmHg.
5. Assure that the scale on the monitor that is connected to the pressure line is at either 0–25 mmHg or 0–50 mmHg to assess diastolic readings upon catheter insertion.
6. Prepare sterile field.
7. Maintain aseptic technique throughout procedure.
8. Label medications to be used.
9. Position patient either flat with minimal Trendelenburg, for superior insertion approach, or supine, for inferior insertion approach.
10. Level transducer with the phlebostatic axis.
11. Turn patient's head away from site and prepare insertion site using aseptic technique.
12. Assist physician with PPE.
13. Once the catheter package is opened, maintaining sterility, the physician will hand off lumen ends.
14. The physician will inflate the balloon, prior to catheter insertion, to ensure function.
15. Flush the lumen ends. The sterile syringes may be left attached, if instructed by the physician.
16. Attach the distal PA lumen end to a monitored pressure line.
17. The physician will insert the introducer that supports the PA catheter after obtaining venous access.
18. The physician, or advanced practice nurse, must change sterile gloves after introducer insertion, before the PA catheter is placed. An additional sterile field should also be applied at this time.

19. The catheter is inserted through the introducer.
20. Monitor closely for arrhythmias and ventricular dys-rhythmias as the catheter is inserted.
21. Waveforms are assessed as the catheter is inserted. Record the pressures:
    a. *Junction of the superior vena cava and right atrium (RA):* An oscillation indicative of respirations is observed. The balloon is inflated.
    b. *RA/central venous pressure (CVP):* A small waveform; normally ranging from 2 to 6 mmHg. This pressure is read in mean.
    c. *Right ventricle (RV):* 15–28/0–8 mmHg with sharp systolic upstrokes and low diastolic dips. Only measured during insertion, indicative of RV, pulmonic, and tricuspid valve function.
    d. *PA:* A smooth upstroke with a systolic pressure near that of the RV. A dicrotic notch on the diastolic stroke is noted, indicating pulmonic valve closure. PA systolic is 15–30 mmHg. It is the pressure in the PA during RV contraction. PA diastolic (PAD) is 5–15 mmHg. It is the resistance of the pulmonary vasculature to blood flow and indirectly measures the left ventricular end-diastolic pressure (LVEDP).
    e. *PAWP:* Normally 4–12 mmHg. The balloon (a 1.5 cc syringe is attached to the balloon port) is inflated and wedges into a small, distal portion of the PA. This occludes the RV and PAD pressures, and, more accurately than PAD, indirectly measures LVEDP. A small waveform is noted. PAWP is read in mean.
22. The balloon is deflated and the catheter drifts back into the PA.
23. A chest x-ray is taken to confirm proper catheter location.

(Adapted from Alexander, 2006; Alspach, 2006; Chohan & Munden, 2007; Ehlers, 2007; Nettina, 2010; Paunovic & Sharma, 2010; Stillwell, 2006; Swan Ganz Catheterization, 2010; Wyckoff et al., 2009.)

Obtaining a CO reading, which is frequently performed using room-temperature injectate versus iced, from a PA catheter, is completed by:

1. Confirming the right computation constant (noted on the catheter package or insert).
2. Smoothly, for less than 4 seconds, injecting 10 cc of facility-specified injectate into the proximal port of the PA catheter. A smooth, even upstroke should be noted on the monitor tracing.
3. Repeating the process a total of three times, the average of which is said to be the CO.

(Adapted from Chohan & Munden, 2007; Ehlers, 2007; Nettina, 2010; Paunovic & Sharma, 2010; Stillwell, 2006; Swan Ganz Catheterization, 2010.)

The monitor measures the CO reading and calculates CI, SVR, and LVSWI, along with several other hemodynamic values, when properly programmed with the correct patient information, such as height and weight. Some PA catheters have the capacity to monitor continuous CO with the use of a thermistor that senses changes in blood temperature and a special monitoring module.

Certain PA catheters have the ability to obtain SvO_2. Prior to sample aspiration, confirm the facility-specified syringe used for this procedure. The blood is drawn from the distal lumen. Ensure that the balloon is deflated during the entire process. Aspirate the sample smoothly and slowly—slower than 1 cc/20 seconds. After blood withdrawal, note the return of a PA waveform.

See Appendix D for normal PA catheter pressures and hemodynamics values. These values will fluctuate according to the patient, medical treatments, and complications.

===== *FAST FACTS in a NUTSHELL*

Complications of PA catheter insertion and monitoring include air embolus, balloon rupture, bundle branch blocks, catheter migration, clots, dysrhythmias, electric shock, infection, hemorrhage, PA infarction, PA perforation, pneumothorax, and vein damage.

Guidelines to obtain proper pressure readings and troubleshoot problems include the following:

- Zero the transducer each shift and as needed.
- Re-level the transducer with the phlebostatic axis when the patient is moved or transported.
- Record catheter pressures at end expiration.
- Inflate the balloon for PAWP slowly and stop when the waveform is noted.
- Do not leave the PA balloon inflated for longer than 15 seconds.
- Do not inflate the balloon beyond the amount recommended by the manufacturer. The maximum inflation is written on the catheter shaft. It is usually 1.5 cc.
- Observe for normal PA waveform post-PAWP.
- Use aseptic technique whenever accessing a PA catheter.
- Note that the correct scale is chosen when monitoring pressures, for example, 40 mmHg scale for PA monitoring.
- Replace cables, tubing, and disposable transducers as needed.
- Observe for air bubbles in the system; remove if noted. Do not flush the air toward the patient.
- Perform dressing changes every 72 hours, and as needed, using aseptic technique.
- Balloon should be inflated if the tip of the catheter is repositioned by an advanced practitioner.
- If a spontaneous wedge waveform is noted, ask the patient to cough—or reposition him or her. Notify the physician if wedge continues.
- Notify the physician, stat, for ventricular dysrhythmias or blood--brain barrier development. Anticipate the repositioning or removal of the catheter.
- Balloon rupture may be present if no resistance is felt during inflation, no wedge waveform occurs, or bleeding is noted in the balloon port. Discontinue use of this port. Notify the physician.

- Maintain the pressure in the pressure bag high enough to allow for a flush rate of 2–3 cc/hour. The pressure must be above the patient's systolic BP for this to occur.
- *Overdampened waveform (no dicrotic notch noted):* Check that connections are secure. Check the flush/pressure bag, ensuring adequate fluid reserve and proper pressure. Remove kinks noted in the excess external catheter length. Aspirate blood from the catheter and flush the system, away from patient. Notify the physician if the problem persists.
- *Abnormal low pressures:* Re-level the transducer and re-zero. If pressures remain low, titrate vasoactive medications, as ordered, and/or notify the physician.
- *No pressure readings:* Check the stopcock position. Ensure that it is turned open to the transducer and the catheter. Check connections.

(Adapted from Alexander, 2006; Alspach, 2006; Chohan & Munden, 2007; Ehlers, 2007; Nettina, 2010; Paunovic & Sharma, 2010; Stillwell, 2006; Swan Ganz Catheterization, 2010; Wyckoff et al., 2009.)

The steps involved in removing a PA catheter are as follows:

1. Educate patient/family.
2. Ensure balloon deflation.
3. Place patient in Trendelenburg position. Turn the patient's head away from the site, if applicable.
4. Turn the stopcock to the off position and disconnect the transducer.
5. Put on PPE.
6. With patient holding breath or on end expiration, pull back the catheter smoothly and swiftly, while observing the EKG monitor. If resistance is noted, stop and call the physician stat.
7. Note intact catheter tip.
8. If the introducer is maintained, place a cap over the catheter insertion site or insert an obturator.

9. If the introducer is to be removed, discard dressing and remove any sutures.
10. Put on new gloves.
11. Remove the introducer in one smooth, swift movement. Note intact tip.
12. Apply pressure to site until hemostasis. This may take 15 minutes or more.
13. Apply a sterile, occlusive dressing.
14. Document the procedure and patient tolerance.
15. Continue to monitor the site frequently for bleeding and/or hematoma.

(Adapted from Alspach, 2006; Chohan & Munden, 2007; Ehlers, 2007; Mobile Infirmary Medical Center, n.d.; Nettina, 2010; Stillwell, 2006; Swan Ganz Catheterization, 2010.)

12

Discussing Dialysis and Continuous Renal Replacement Therapy

INTRODUCTION

Dialysis is simply the migration of molecules from an area of higher concentration to one of lower concentration through a semi-permeable membrane. Sometimes osmosis is involved. Being such a straightforward action, it might seem strange that so many issues surrounding dialysis exist. Hemodialysis is probably the most common form of dialysis, but continuous renal replacement therapy (CRRT) and peritoneal dialysis are closing in fast.

It has been proven that the sooner dialysis is started, the better the outcome for the patient. Determining the need for dialysis can be tedious and many problems can occur from this "simple" procedure, especially when critically ill patients are concerned.

In this chapter you will learn:

1. The definition, function, and complications related to the different types of dialysis.

2. The variations of CRRT and troubleshooting tips.
3. The types of dialysis vascular access devices (VADs) and proper care instructions.

DIALYSIS

Patients suffering from a number of ailments require dialysis. Issues considered before dialysis initiation include: acute versus chronic renal failure, effectiveness of current medical and pharmacological therapy, electrolyte balance, acidosis status, toxicities, blood urea nitrogen (BUN), and creatinine. **The forms of dialysis vary in capacity to remove excess fluid, waste, medications, and electrolytes.** When caring for a patient undergoing dialysis, it is important to know whether their medications are dialyzable and adjust dosing appropriately, especially antibiotics.

════════════════════════════════FAST FACTS in a NUTSHELL

Dialysis is not a kidney replacement; only some excretory functions are restored. None of the endocrine or metabolic functions of the kidney are simulated.

Patients receiving dialysis require education and emotional support. The constant connection to a machine can be daunting. Diets are restricted, and hospital staff should practice re-enforcement.

Itchy, dry, flaky skin is a common complaint related to ongoing changes in fluid and electrolyte balance. Facility-approved lotion and gentle cleansing with mild soap greatly improves this condition. Patients should be turned and re-positioned every 2 hours to maintain skin integrity.

HEMODIALYSIS

As previously mentioned, dialysis revolves around diffusion and osmosis. Ultrafiltration and convection are also involved.

These actions involve the movement of molecules through a semipermeable membrane via the use of hydrostatic pressure. This is how hemodialysis (HD) works.

Central vascular access is obtained and blood is moved through an external dialyzer, then returned to the body, all by a blood pump. **The dialyzer contains a semipermeable membrane that filters out toxins, waste, metabolic by-products, excess fluid, and so on.**

HD can be long- or short-term. Patients without risk of hemorrhage receive heparin, according to facility protocol and individual needs. **Central vascular access varies based on the patient, situation, and expected term of HD.** Frequency of treatment is usually every day for the first several days, then 3 times a week but can differ according to necessity. The duration of each HD session is approximately 2 to 4 hours. It may occur at the bedside or in a dialysis unit and is frequently performed by specially trained dialysis nurses and technicians.

HD is contraindicated for patients with labile hemodynamics and/or problems surrounding heparin. **Patients in the ICU are often too unstable to tolerate HD** because it involves the movement of approximately 300 ml of blood at any given time, along with major shifts in fluid and electrolytes.

═══════════════════════════════*FAST FACTS in a NUTSHELL*

Complications related to HD are altered level of consciousness, anaphylaxis, angina, bleeding, EKG changes, electrolyte imbalance, fever, hemolysis, hypotension, hypertension, hypovolemia, infection, muscle cramps, nausea, and vomiting.

Patients suffering from a drug overdose or exposure to toxins, such as bromide, chloral hydrate, ethanol, ethylene glycol, lithium, methanol, or salicylate **can be treated with HD.** It is initiated within 4 to 6 hours of exposure or ingestion, if possible.

Continuous Renal Replacement Therapy

CCRT is a type of dialysis designed with the critical care patient in mind. The amount of blood used at one time is much smaller. The treatment occurs 24 hours a day, 7 days a week. These two factors reduce extreme changes in the level of circulating fluid volume, toxins, waste, electrolytes, etc. CRRT involves the use of a porous filter and an extracorporeal blood circuit.

CRRT is ideal for patients with unstable hemodynamics, pulmonary edema, or acute myocardial infarction requiring dialysis. The only contraindication to CRRT is an extremely elevated hematocrit (Hct): Hct >45. Such patients are often still able to receive certain forms of dialysis, such as continuous venovenous hemofiltration.

There are several types of CCRT:

- *Slow continuous ultrafiltration (SCUF):* Uses heparin; involves ultrafiltration and an effluent pump to control the ultrafiltration rate. Requires arteriovenous (AV) access; often used for removing large amounts of fluid.
- *Continuous arteriovenous hemofiltration (CAVH):* Uses heparin; requires an AV site. Functions similarly to SCUF with like exchange variables; replacement fluid is used. Mean arterial pressure (MAP) should be at least 60 mmHg.
- *Continuous arteriovenous hemodialysis (CAVHD):* Uses heparin; is CAVH combined with HD. Aided by a pump, dialysate flows in the oppsite direction of the blood, allowing diffusion and convection to occur. Fluid and molecules are removed with this method.
- *Continuous venovenous hemofiltration (CVVH):* Seen frequently in ICU; requires anticoagulation. Uses a dual-lumen venovenous access, a blood pump and an electrolyte- or sodium bicarbonate-based replacement fluid. Involves ultrafiltration and convection. Removes fluid and molecules.
- *Continuous venovenous hemodialysis (CVVHD):* Uses heparin or trisodium citrate (closely monitor Ca+

levels). Involves ultrafiltration, diffusion, and osmosis. Requires dual-lumen venovenous access, blood pump and dialysate, flowing in the opposite direction of the blood. No replacement fluid is needed.

- *Continuous venovenous hemodiafiltration (CVVHDF):* Uses heparin or trisodium citrate (closely moniotr Ca+ levels). Requires a dual-lumen venovenous access site, blood pump, and dialysate, flowing in the opposite direction of the blood. Involves convection and diffusion. Replacement fluid is necessary. Capable of moving high volumes of fluid hourly.

(Adapted from Alspach, 2006; Chohan & Munden, 2007; Ehlers, 2007; Mobile Medical Infirmary Unit, n.d.; Nettina, 2010; Stillwell, 2006.)

CVVH and CVVHDF are the most frequently used forms of CRRT. These methods provide a more consistent blood flow rate than do others.

═══════════════════════════════*FAST FACTS in a NUTSHELL*

How Blood Flows to Complete CVVHDF:

1. Blood is pulled at 200 ml/hour by a blood pump from the venovenous access catheter.
2. Heparin and fluid are mixed with the blood.
3. The solution is pushed through a hemofilter/dialyzer, the semipermeable membrane that removes waste.
4. At the same time, ultrafiltrate is pulled into the collection bag.
5. The blood/solution then goes through a drip chamber to remove air and clots. It passes through a bubble detector, where a clamp closes the system if air is found.
6. The blood/solution is returned to the patient.

(Adapted from Alspach, 2006; Chohan & Munden, 2007; Ehlers, 2007; Mobile Medical Infirmary Unit, n.d.; Nettina, 2010; Stillwell, 2006.)

Employing CRRT at the bedside requires several steps:

1. Verify physician's order and patient identity via two identifiers.
2. Obtain CRRT machine and required supplies.
3. Review lab results, such as electrolytes, clotting times and factors, ABGs, hemogram, BUN, and creatinine.
4. Note vital signs, hemodynamics, and patient weight.
5. Give ordered bolus of heparin.
6. Educate patient and family.
7. Prime dialyzer and tubing lines per facility/manufacturer guidelines.
8. Follow facility guidelines regarding the preparation of the vascular access device (VAD)/catheter lumens for CRRT applications.
9. Follow facility/manufacturer guidelines pertaining to the preparation of connection sites prior to attaching to catheter ports/lumens.
10. Using aseptic technique, securely connect the dialyzer circuit to vascular access site(s).
11. Set blood pump rate.
12. Set air and venous pressure-detecting equipment.
13. Start dialysate, if applicable.
14. Begin replacement fluid infusion, if ordered.
15. Observe blood flow rate through the tubing.
16. When a gravity collection bag is used, keep it at least 16 inches below the dialyzer.
17. Titrate settings according to patient tolerance.
18. Assess machine, circuit, and tubing for leaks, disconnections, and clotting.
19. Frequently assess access site
20. If monitoring a femoral VAD, palpate pulses hourly. Assess for discolored skin, a cool extremity, and pain at site. The patient should not bend legs more than 30° at the hips.
21. Record total patient input/output hourly, including amount of fluid in collection bag and insensible losses.
22. Continually monitor vital signs, EKG, and hemodynamics.
23. Monitor ultrafiltrate (the fluid in collection bag). It should be clear or slightly yellow. Pink or bloody color

may indicate a dialyzer leak; call MD and anticipate stopping CRRT. For CVVH, the blood-leak detector signals an alert that indicates a leak.

24. If pressure alarms sound, check the corresponding catheter/tubing/port for kinks, blockages, and disconnections.
25. Items to note and record include:
    a. Access pressure, venous pressure, and effluent pressure.
    b. Replacement fluid/dialysate rate.
    c. Blood flow rate.
    d. Patient fluid removal rate.
    e. Calculated hourly filtrate rate.
    f. Actual ultrafiltrate volume.
    g. Cumulative total of patient fluid removed.

Troubleshooting guidelines pertaining to CRRT include:

- For a decrease in B/P, place the patient flat or in Trendelenburg position. Slow the ultrafiltrate rate. Give a small normal saline bolus or a vasoactive drug; administer replacement fluid, if ordered.
- For continued low B/P, clamp ultrafiltrate tubing and call MD immediately.
- When a gravity collection bag is used, the ultrafiltrate rate can be adjusted by changing the distance between the dialyzer and the collection bag. Raising the bed to increase distance may increase flow. Lowering the bed to decrease distance may slow flow.
- When a blood pump is used, ultrafiltrate rate can be adjusted by changing the blood pump rate.
- For decreased ultrafiltrate output, check the system and access site for kinks. Assess dialyzer for clots. Assess for lowered patient blood flow indicated by a decrease in hemodynamics.
- For decreased ultrafiltrate output accompanied by dark blood in the circuit or an increase in venous pressure during CVVH, check the filter. It might be clotted. Anticipate changing the entire circuit.

- Patients receiving an ACE inhibitor could be at an increased risk for an allergic reaction to chemicals that come in contact with the filter used in some CRRT dialyzers. Assess the patient and notify MD PRN.

(Adapted from Alspach, 2006; Chohan & Munden, 2007; Ehlers, 2007; McDemott, 2009; Mobile Infirmary Medical Center, n.d.; Nettina, 2010; Stillwell, 2006; University of Connecticut Health Center, 2009.)

It is recommended that a flow rate of 50 ml/min for approximately 10 minutes during CRRT initiation be maintained. The flow can then be increased 25 ml/min each minute until the physician-ordered rate is met. If the patient's vital signs or hemodynamics change, reduce flow rate and call the physician.

CRRT orders are renewed daily and adjusted to the patient's current status. **Closely monitor the patient's body temperature**, along with other vital signs, as heat is lost as the blood is circulated through the extracorporeal region of the CRRT circuit.

==*FAST FACTS in a NUTSHELL*

Complications that can occur with CRRT include: air embolus, bleeding, clotting, electrolyte imbalance, fluid imbalance, hypotension, infection, and thrombosis.

PERITONEAL DIALYSIS

Peritoneal dialysis **(PD) is not frequently used in the ICU.** If patients are unable to tolerate HD, CRRT is generally the dialysis method of choice. However, PD is a viable dialysis option for several medical issues. It works via osmosis and diffusion. Protein loss and minimal ability to remove potassium are two disadvantages. The contraindications to PD are abdominal adhesions, bleeding disorders, and recent peritoneal surgery.

During PD, a warmed (98.6°F) dialysate, consisting of hypertonic glucose, is instilled into the peritoneal cavity via a catheter. Aseptic technique is practiced. The fluid is instilled for at least 30 minutes, then drained by gravity over about 15 minutes. This continuous cycle is repeated per physician order; dwell time may last as long as 4 days.

Very little heparin is needed for this form of dialysis, and there is minimal affect on hemodynamics. Heparin, insulin, and/or antibiotics may be added to the dialysate, using sterile technique.

Assess the abdomen for pain and tenderness. If abdominal pain is encountered during instillation, slow the infusion. Monitor the effluent (drainage from catheter). It should be straw colored. Notify the physician of changes in color, clarity, and fibrin particles. Measure the amount of effluent removed.

If draining effluent becomes slow, check for tubing kinks and clamping. Try to turn the patient side to side, elevate the head of the bed, adjust the drainage bag lower, and apply light pressure to the abdomen. If effluent still will not drain, call the physician immediately.

Until the catheter site is healed, sterile dressing changes are performed daily and PRN. Once healed, the site is washed gently with soap and water. An antibiotic ointment or iodine solution application follows.

════════════════════════*FAST FACTS in a NUTSHELL*

Possible complications related to PD include: bladder or bowel perforation, bleeding, peritonitis, and respiratory distress caused by increased abdominal girth.

VASCULAR ACCESS DEVICES

Every form of dialysis, except PD, requires a vascular access device (VAD). There are several types of VADs. The type used varies with the form of dialysis, length of treatment expected, urgency of dialysis, and individual patient characteristics.

Central venous access is performed for emergency situations and as a bridge to permanent catheter placement/ repair. A double- or triple-lumen catheter is inserted, using aseptic technique, into the internal jugular, subclavian, or femoral vein by an advanced practioner.

The temporary VAD site should be frequently assessed for bleeding, hematoma, dislodgement, and kinking. For femoral vein access, palpate peripheral pulses during assessments. Sterile dressing changes should occur every 48 hours and PRN.

Lumen catheters and ports should be accessed using aseptic technique. Heparinizing them is done according to manufacturer/facility protocol. If heparin is instilled in the lumen catheter, ensure that the appropriate amount of fluid is withdrawn and wasted before flushing or connecting dialysis circuits. Do not use a VAD to administer medications, IV fluids, or blood products except with a written physician/advanced practitioner order in emergency situations where the patient has no other vascular access.

Permanent vascular access is commonly achieved with an AV fistula in the upper arm. This procedure is completed in the OR with an anastomosis of an artery and vein or an artificial graft.

═════════════════════════*FAST FACTS in a NUTSHELL*

Guidelines to follow when caring for a patient with an AV fistula:

- Always perfrom hand hygiene before touching the site.
- A thrill should be palpable over the fistula, indicating patency.
- A bruit should be heard over the fistula, indicating patency.
- Venipuncture, IV access, injections, and blood pressure readings are not performed on the affected arm.
- Circumferential dressings are not applied to the affected arm.
- Assess the site for skin-color changes, bleeding, redness, bulging, warmth, edema, and drainage.
- Assess capillary refill and sensation.

(Adapted from Alexander, 2006; Nettina, 2010; Rushing, 2010.)

FAST FACTS in a NUTSHELL

Complications related to an AV fistula include: aneurysm, clotting, infection, ischemia of the hand, stenosis, and thrombosis.

An external AV shunt is an option for vascular access but is seldom used. It requires the use of a sterile dressing and daily dressing changes. Otherwise, care and assessment is similar to that of an AV fistula site. Clotting is a major problem with this type of device.

13

Cardiac Specialty Equipment

INTRODUCTION

The equipment used in the ICU often differs from that throughout the rest of a hospital. In the cardiac unit, equipment is often more disease-specific. A temporary pacemaker, intra-aortic balloon pump (IABP), and left-ventricular assist device (LVAD) are examples of equipment that cardiac ICU nurses should be proficient in operating. While identified in this chapter as cardiac specific, these devices may be used in other ICUs.

In this chapter you will learn:

1. The ins and outs of a temporary pacemaker and an IABP.
2. The various types of ventricular assist devices.
3. Troubleshooting guidelines for cardiac equipment.

TEMPORARY PACEMAKER

Implementation of a temporary pacemaker occurs frequently in the ICU. The transcutaneous approach, involving pacing pads placed on the external chest wall connected to a defibrillator with a pacing mechanism, is temporary, and it can be painful. It is usually reserved for emergency situations. Other modes of pacing include internal or endocardial leads, atrial or ventricular epicardial leads placed at the time of surgery, transcutaneous insertion via a needle placed directly through the chest wall, and an esophageal electrode used for atrial pacing and recording.

Like permanent pacemakers, **temporary pacemakers cause the myocardium of the heart to depolarize, causing a muscle "contraction."** This occurs easily in healthy heart tissue. However, patients with cardiac problems may not conform easily. Fine-tuning is necessary to assure proper device function.

A transvenous pacemaker is placed in the right ventricle, for a single-chamber device, or into the right atrium and right ventricle for a dual chamber device. The subclavian, internal jugular, antecubital, or femoral vein allows access. Insertion of a temporary pacemaker is an aseptic procedure that can be performed at the bedside, if needed, by an advanced practioner. A pacing catheter is inserted and its pacing wire connected to a programmable, external generator that is often referred to as a pacemaker box. Refer to Chapter 9 for central venous line insertion, care, and removal guidelines.

Epicardial wires, inserted during coronary artery bypass graft surgery, can be used for temporary pacing. The wires are attached to the myocardium, then tunneled out through the chest wall. The appropriate positive and negative poles are connected to an external generator and the ordered settings initiated.

If not in use, epicardial wires usually remain in place for approximately 48 hours post-op. A sterile occlusive dressing protects the site. It is changed each day or per facility protocol. When it is time for removal, the procedure is completed, at the bedside, by an advanced practioner.

The major components of a temporary pacemaker are the box and the leads. The box, or pulse generator, is powered by batteries and has dials that are set to control the function of the device. The lead(s) relays the information from the generator to the heart tissue. These wires are actually positive and negative electrodes. Each is placed in the corresponding hole when connecting the leads to the cable that attaches to the generator.

A pacemaker can pace via the atria, the ventricle, or both. Pacing spikes on EKG tracings provide evidence of this; refer to Appendix B for an example.

Sensing is a pacemaker feature that detects natural cardiac activity that is not machine generated. It is set via the generator, or box. There are three categories: demand, fixed, and triggered. Demand allows the device to sense intrinsic activity and provide only those beats needed to maintain a pre-set heart rate. A fixed setting has no sensing capacity; a certain amount of beats will be provided regardless of the underlying rhythm. Lastly, triggered sensing allows the device to pick up intrinsic cardiac activity and adjust accordingly. This type of sensing may be in response to atrial activity, cardiac muscle activity, temperature changes, oxygen consumption, or blood pH.

Capture is the pacemaker's capability to create a contraction after it delivers an electrical impulse to the tissue. It is observed on an EKG when a P wave, or QRS, immediately follows a pacing spike. Refer to Appendix B for an example.

To confirm proper pacemaker function, most devices have a sense indicator light that flashes with each heartbeat. Palpation of a pulse correlating with the EKG tracing is also confirmation of pacemaker capture.

═══════════════════════════════*FAST FACTS in a NUTSHELL*

Milliamperes (mA) is the unit in which pacemaker output is measured. Usually, capture is "found" at 5 to 20 mA for atrial leads and 5 to 25 mA for ventricular leads. Upon initial set-up, output is generally set at 5 mA and lowered until capture is lost (noted on the EKG). The output is then programmed and maintained at 2 to 3 times the minimum level required for capture. If capture is lost at a higher level, the output is programmed and maintained 2 to 3 mA higher than that level to prevent pacing wire burnout.

The rate for a temporary pacemaker is usually set between 60 and 80 beats per minute. With a properly functioning device, the EKG should be scoping at or above,the set rate of the pacemaker, when in the demand mode. Cardiac monitors should be programmed to recognize pacing to avoid double counting the patient's heart rate.

It is important to become familiar with the function and dials of the pacemaker generator utilized in each facility, prior to the need for one. Several companies manufacture temporary pacing devices, while all work similarly, appearances and dial locations vary.

An advanced practitioner orders initial settings for a temporary pacemaker. If loss of capture, failure to sense, or alterations in the patient's condition occur, the settings can be adjusted.

Patients receiving temporary pacemaker therapy require constant EKG monitoring. Changes in the EKG tracing, hemodynamics, or overall assessment should be reported to the physician immediately.

═══════════════════════════*FAST FACTS in a NUTSHELL*

Complications related to temporary pacemaker placement and usage include: arrhythmia, bleeding, pericardial effusion, cardiac tamponade, device malfunction, embolus, heart failure, hemothorax, infection, lead migration, pain, pneumothorax, thrombus, and diaphragmic twitching (hiccups) with device-delivered electrical impulses.

Nursing interventions that may prevent complications related to temporary pacemaker placement and usage include:

• Closely monitor EKG tracing. Ensure the detection of pacing spikes, set appropriate alarms, and confirm that they are on.

- Assess EKG for pacer spikes occurring too close to the T-wave. Prevent R-on-T phenomenon, potentially causing V-tach, by adjusting settings or turn off the device and notify the MD. Apply and use external pacing pads, if needed.
- Ensure that a post-insertion chest x-ray has been taken and read.
- Feel for palpable pulse with each noted QRS.
- Perform frequent patient assessments, including:
  a. Vital signs and hemodynamics.
  b. Level of consciousness.
  c. Breath sounds.
  d. Skin color and perfusion.
  e. Capillary refill.
  f. Urinary output.
  g. Jaw or ear pain; may indicate catheter migration.
- Notify MD of changes, PRN.
- Monitor insertion site for bleeding.
- Palpate distal pulses frequently.
- Monitor for changes in electrolytes, myocardial function, and O_2 levels.
- Properly secure leads and pacing catheter.
- Use adequate staff and maneuvering to transfer and re-position patient to prevent lead dislodgement.
- Change dressing on insertion site every 72 hours and PRN, using aseptic technique
- Wear rubber gloves when touching pacing wires.
- Protect exposed parts of the leads, as recommended by manufacturer.
- Maintain the clear, hard, plastic protective covering over the generator to prevent an accidental change in settings.
- If the patient has epicardial wires that are not connected, the ends should be placed in a plastic tube and the tube put in a rubber glove for protection.
- Make sure all equipment is grounded with a three-prong plug.
- Do not allow the use of electric razors.

- Be aware that electrocautery and transcutaneous electrical stimulators can interfere with temporary pacemaker function.
- Always recheck pacemaker function after defibrillation/cardioversion.
- Be prepared to administer atropine and/or isoproterenol in case of device failure.
- Provide patient and family education.
- Encourage cough and deep breathe every 2 hours.
- Perform ROM every 2 hours, if possible.

(Adapted from Alspach, 2006; Chohan & Munden, 2007; Ehlers, 2007; Nettina, 2010; Stillwell, 2006.)

═══════════════════════*FAST FACTS in a NUTSHELL*

Troubleshooting Tips for Temporary Pacemakers

- *Failure to capture:* Check the battery. Secure connections box, leads, and the patient. Increase MA. Re-position patient to left side. Rule out conditions such as hyperkalemia or acidosis that may cause reduced myocardial response. Prepare to externally pace if unable to resolve.
- *Failure to sense:* Check battery and connections. Increase sensitivity settings by lowering the millivolts. Turn patient onto left side.
- *Hypotension:* Increase pacemaker rate. Rule out other causes.

INTRA-AORTIC BALLOON PUMP

An intra-aortic balloon (IAB) is inserted to assist a heart that is not functioning properly. It provides afterload reduction to impaired ventricles and added perfusion to the coronaries, brain, and kidneys with the use of a sausage-shaped, helium-filled balloon that rests in the descending aorta distal to the left subclavian artery and proximal to the renal arteries. Arterial access, via the femoral artery, is usually obtained in a cardiac catheterization lab (CCL) using fluoroscopy.

═══════════════════════════*FAST FACTS in a NUTSHELL*

An IAB is employed for a variety of medical issues, including acute myocardial infarction, multiple types of shock, papillary muscle malfunctions, unstable angina, and ventricular defects. Contraindications for its use are an aortic aneurysm, aortic insufficiency, aortic calcification or vegetation, coagulopathy, end-stage terminal illness, grafts in the thoracic aorta, and peripheral vascular disease.

An IAB is a catheter with a balloon tip that connects to a computer and monitor that controls the balloon's function, which is referred to as counterpulsation. The intra-aortic balloon pump (IABP) works when the cardiac muscle rests, and it rests when the cardiac muscle contracts.

The balloon inflates at the start of diastole, during aortic valve closure (as depicted by the dicrotic notch on the arterial BP waveform) and quickly **deflates just before systole,** when the aortic valve opens. A sharp V is noted in the waveform. **The proper timing of inflation and deflation is important because it allows maximum perfusion assistance and provides lower pressures for ventricle emptying.** Thus, timing is constantly monitored.

Early inflation of the balloon can cause aortic regurgitation, early aortic valve closure, increases in afterload, LVEDP/PCWP, and myocardial oxygen consumption (MVO_2). It is evidenced by inflation of the balloon prior to the dicrotic notch.

Late inflation can cause poor coronary perfusion. It is characterized by balloon inflation after the dicrotic notch, no sharp V wave, and poor diastolic augmentation. A W-shaped waveform is often noted.

Early deflation can cause poor coronary perfusion, retrograde coronary/carotid flow, chest pain, poor afterload reduction, and increased MVO_2. The augmented waveform will have a sharp drop (U shape) after diastolic augmentation and/or reduced diastolic augmentation. The assisted and unassisted aortic end-diastolic pressures may be equal. The assisted systolic pressure could rise.

Late deflation leads to almost no afterload reduction. The balloon is inflated for too long. MVO_2, afterload, and preload are all at risk for increase. This is a peak systolic pressure that exceeds assisted peak systolic pressure.

The trigger of an IABP is usually the EKG, and the timing is dialed in according to the arterial BP waveform. The IABP can be set to augment with every cardiac cycle, every other cycle, or every third or fourth cycle.

EKG electrodes from the IABP are placed on the patient's chest or "slaved" from an existing EKG monitor into the machine. **Lead II is generally the best choice for monitoring** because the R wave is often easily seen in this lead. The lead position showing the biggest R wave is needed because the R wave commonly triggers the IABP.

Most IABPs can also be set to automatically inflate with the dicrotic notch or the middle of the T-wave. **Newer systems have a one-button start key and automatically adjust to changes in patient status.**

Proper balloon size is needed for optimal IAB augmentation. Size is chosen based on the patient's height and is noted by the manufacturer on the balloon catheter packaging.

═══════════════════════════════════════ *FAST FACTS in a NUTSHELL*

Several factors may lead to poor IABP augmentation such as increased heart rate, poor balloon position, reduced hemodynamics, wrong balloon size, and wrong timing. Complications related to an IABP include: aortic aneurysm rupture, aortic dissection, arterial obstruction, arterial perforation, atelectasis, compartment syndrome, embolus, infection, hematoma, hemorrhage, thrombocytopenia, and thrombus.

Several interventions are implemented when caring for a patient with an IABP:

- Frequent assessment of:
  1. Vital signs and EKG
  2. Hemodynamics
  3. Urine output
  4. Level of consciousness and neuro components
  5. Peripheral pulses: pedal, post-tibial, radial, and brachial
  6. Insertion site
  7. Balloon augmentation
  8. Pain
  9. Bowel sounds
  10. Coagulation lab results
- Secure all connections between pump and patient.
- Immobilize the leg used for IABP.
- Frequently change the patient's position while maintaining IABP-leg immobilization.
- Maintain the head of the bed at 15° to 30°.
- Ensure that balloon inflation is timed at the dicrotic notch and deflation just before the next systole.
- Make adjustments to balloon timing to maximize diastolic augmentation and minimize aortic end-diastolic pressure.
- Use IABP mean arterial pressure (MAP) for titration of vasoactive medications.
- Do not obtain blood samples from the IABP balloon catheter. It increases the risk of thrombus formation.
- Never allow the balloon to be stopped for longer than 30 minutes because of a high risk for thrombus.
- Encourage coughing and deep breathing, along with incentive spirometry.
- Assess and treat pain frequently.
- Change the insertion site dressing every 24 hours and PRN using aseptic technique.
- Provide patient/family education and emotional support.
- Obtain a daily chest x-ray

- Notify MD and anticipate a chest x-ray for questionable balloon placement.

(Adapted from Alspach, 2006; Chohan & Munden, 2007; Datascope, n.d.; Krishna & Zarcharowski, 2009; Mullens, 2008; Nettina, 2010; St. Luke's Episcopal Hospital n.d.; Stillwell, 2006; Wyckoff et al., 2009.)

═══════════════ *FAST FACTS in a NUTSHELL*

Tips for troubleshooting an IABP:
- Evaluate timing in the 1:2 (1 balloon inflation cycle to 2 cardiac cycles) augmentation setting.
- *Atrial fibrillation:* Use automatic timing. Notify MD.
- *Red/brown color noted in balloon connector tubing:* Indicative of balloon leak. The blood detect, low augmentation, gas loss, and/or IABP catheter alarms may also sound. Put IABP in standby mode and call MD. Anticipate device removal.
- *Decrease in urine output, altered LOC, and/or changes in peripheral pulses:* Indicative of balloon migration; notify MD.
- *Complete IABP control console malfunction:* Obtain another console. While waiting for a new console, manually inflate the balloon with a 60-ml syringe, using room air, every 5 minutes.
- *Gas leak alarm:* Check all connections and for water condensation in the IABP tubing. Could indicate a balloon leak. Notify MD.

Several factors can cause the balloon waveform on the IABP console to change in appearance:
- Bradycardia: longer plateau, wider waveform.
- Tachycardia: shorter plateau, thinner waveform.
- Irregular heart rhythm: varying waveform widths.
- Hypotension: shorter waveform.
- Hypertension: taller waveform.
- Gas loss/leak in IABP system: waveform dips below baseline tracing.
- Catheter kink: waveform is rounded on the top.

(Adapted from Alspach, 2006; Chohan & Munden, 2007; Datascope, n.d.; Krishna & Zarcharowski, 2009; Mullens, 2008; Nettina, 2010; St. Luke's Episcopal Hospital n.d.; Stillwell, 2006; Wyckoff et al., 2009.)

A weaning process is completed before an IAB is removed. The frequency of augmentation is reduced to 1:2, then 1:3, then 1:4 as tolerated, per physician parameters. The **1:3 or 1:4 ratio should not be used for longer than 2 hours prior to balloon removal** because of the potentional for thrombus formation.

An IAB can be discontinued, at the bedside, by an advanced practioner. **After the balloon and catheter are removed, the site must be closely monitored.** Pressure is applied until hemostasis, often 30 minutes or more, followed by either a pressure dressing or sandbag. Hematoma, bleeding, and retroperitoneal bleeding are possible. **Check the site frequently and thoroughly.** Bed rest is required for 24 hours post-IAB removal.

VENTRICULAR ASSIST DEVICE

A ventricular assist device (VAD) gives support to a poorly functioning, or failing, heart while providing perfusion to the rest of the body. **Its primary function is to reduce the cardiac workload and increase the output.** A VAD is frequently used as a bridge to a heart transplant. It is also inserted temporarily to assist with the weaning of cardiopulmonary bypass or as support during recovery from cardiogenic shock.

The basic mechanism of a VAD revolves around an artificial pump and its essential function as a ventricle. Blood is diverted from the patient's failing ventricle to the pump, which pushes the blood out to the aorta or pulmonary system. This action is synchronized with the cardiac cycle using an EKG. A VAD is inserted in the OR or CCL.

There are several types of VADs. A right VAD supports the pulmonary system when the right ventricle fails. A left VAD helps a weakened left ventricle supply blood to the body via the aorta. A combination of the two is a biventricular (BiVAD) device.

VADs can be classified by functionality type. There are resuscitative devices, such as cardiopulmonary bypass and an extracorpeal (outside the body) membrane oxygenation system, external nonpulsatile devices, such as the Bio-Medicus, external pulsatile assist devices, such as the ABIOMED 5000 and Thoratec VAD, and implantable VADs, such as the HeartMate.

============================= *FAST FACTS in a NUTSHELL*

Potential complications resulting from the use of VAD therapy include an air embolus, arrhythmias, failure of the unassisted ventricle, infection, hemorrhage, hypoxemia, and thrombus. Few contraindications exist, as this is a last-resort intervention when other treatments have proven unsuccessful and is often a bridge to transplant.

Caring for a patient with a VAD requires several nursing implementations:

- Frequent assessment of:
    1. Vital signs, EKG, and temperature.
    2. Hemodynamics; maintain MAP >70 mmHg, or as ordered.
    3. Peripheral pulses.
    4. Breath sounds.
    5. Level of consciosness and neuro components.
    6. Chest tubes; notify MD if drainage >150 ml/hour for 2 hours.
    7. Insertion site.
    8. Fluid/hydration status.
    9. Urine output.
    10. Pain.
    11. Bowel sounds.
    12. Coagulation lab results.
    13. Hemoglobin and hematocrit.
- Assess for signs and symptoms of bleeding; heparinization is often required.
- Assess for increased jugular venous distension (JVD) and peripheral edema. Notify MD if found.

- Avoid tension and kinking in the device tubing.
- In the situation of cardiac arrest, use advanced cardiac life support protocol (ACLS). Anticipate the use of internal cardiac massage and internal defibrillation.
- Apply blankets PRN; patients tend to have heat loss.
- Complete range-of-motion exercises twice a day, if possible.
- Turn the patient every two hours, if possible.
- Encourage coughing and deep breathing, along with incentive spirometry, if possible.

(Adapted from Alspach, 2006; Chohan & Munden, 2007; Datascope, n.d.; Ehlers, 2007; Krishna & Zarcharowski, 2009; Mullens, 2008; Nettina, 2010; St. Luke's Episcopal Hospital n.d.; Stillwell, 2006; Wyckoff et al., 2009.)

ABIOMED 5000

The ABIOMED 5000 is an example of a VAD that is inserted for short-term therapy. It is an external device, is FDA approved as a bridge to recovery from reversible heart failure (Wyckoff, Houghton, & LePage, 2009), and is used in the hospital. It can be right, left, or biventricular.

The ABIOMED 5000 has an extracorpeal, air-driven pump with a dual-chamber design. An atrial chamber fills with blood via gravity, and a ventricular chamber pumps blood out. Valves separate the chambers. The ventricle chamber is connected to a monitor console. Cannulas are connected from the pump to the patient. Blood flow via this device is up to 5 L per minute. This device is automatic, adjusts to changes in pre-load and after-load, and has the capacity for weaning.

═══════════════════════════*FAST FACTS in a NUTSHELL*

Tips for ABIOMED 5000 console operation and implementation:

- Assure the console is plugged into a three-prong outlet with a ground and emergency generator back-up.

Continued

Continued

- For a 42 French (Fr) atrial cannula, adjust the level of the blood pump between 0 and 10 inches below the level of the atrium.
- For a 32 or 36 Fr atrial cannula, adjust the level of the blood pump between 4 and 14 inches below the level of the atrium.
- Monitor blood chambers for complete filling and draining.
- Assess the valves of the pump chambers, with a flashlight, every 2 hours, for thrombus formation.
- Assess the valves of the "ventricle" every 8 hours for thrombus formation.
- Secure all connections between the cannula, console, and patient.

(Adapted from Alspach, 2006; Chohan & Munden, 2007; Datascope, n.d.; Ehlers, 2007; Nettina, 2010; St. Luke's Episcopal Hospital n.d.; Stillwell, 2006.)

Various alarms may sound from the ABIOMED 5000. Troubleshooting tips follow:

- *Low flow:* Check for line obstruction. Lower the blood pump chamber. Infuse IV fluid or blood, as ordered. If the patient has a LVAD only, employ vasoactive medications to increase right ventricular function, as ordered.
- *Low pressure/low flow:* Assess tubing connections, particularly at the console. Note any leaks in the tubing and replace PRN.
- *High pressure/low flow:* Assess for kinks in the tubing or cannulas. Lower SVR with medications, as prescribed. Maintain SBP <140 mmHg, or as ordered.
- *Low battery:* Plug in the console.
- *Continuous audible alarm:* Use the foot/hand pump to operate the device. Seek help from the ICU staff and MD.
- *Complete failure:* Use the foot/hand pump to operate the VAD. Call for a new console and help.

(Adapted from Alspach, 2006; Chohan & Munden, 2007; Datascope, n.d.; Ehlers, 2007; Nettina, 2010; St. Luke's Episcopal Hospital n.d.; Stillwell, 2006.)

THORATEC VAD

A Thoratec VAD is used in the hospital and can provide right, left, or biventricular support. A blood pump is positioned extracorporeally and connected to cannulas that are inserted into the heart.

The pump is housed in a hard plastic case that holds a flexible pumping bag. Blood is pushed from the pump when the bag is compressed by air that is controlled by an external console. Mechanical valves control the direction of blood flow within the system. The resulting blood flow can be as great as 7 L per minute.

This pulsatile system can be set in one of three modes: asynchronous (pumping occurs at a pre-set rate), synchronous (pumping is synched with the heart rate), or volume (pumping is determined by the LV filling volume). The console monitors, controls, and displays the device's parameters and function.

IMPELLA

The Impella device by ABIOMED is the smallest VAD available at the time of publication. Partial assistance is provided to the ventricle by reducing MVO_2 and increasing cardiac output, along with coronary and organ perfusion.

An Impella is used during high-risk coronary angioplasty and/or stenting procedures. It can be maintained, post-procedure, to provide support until the patient recovers sufficiently to tolerate weaning of the device or until a longer term VAD is placed. Reducing pump performance completes the weaning process.

This VAD is inserted, under fluoroscopy in the CCL, via the femoral artery. The tip of its catheter has a pigtail that rests in the LV and produces blood flow. An Impella is generally monitored by an ICU nurse and maintained by a perfusionist(s).

==*FAST FACTS in a NUTSHELL*

Therapy with an Impella is not recommended for more than 5 to 7 days and several contraindications exist, such as: aortic insufficiency, cardiogenic shock, ST-segment elevation, and myocardial infarction within 3 days or CPR within 24 hours prior to tentative insertion. The cardiologist ultimately determines use.

The Impella console has a similar appearance to that of an IABP and heparinization is used. Refer to manufacturer guidelines for troubleshooting and call the physician, as needed. Maintain immobilization of the leg used for device insertion. Practice the general nursing implementations for patients undergoing VAD therapy.

PORTABLE VADS

Certain VADs allow patients to be discharged from the hospital and resume the activities of daily life. These devices are small, functional, and an important part of heart-failure treatment.

Patients using these devices require extensive education and emotional support, as well as frequent medical follow-up. Because they are used at home, troubleshooting guidelines are not provided here. Refer to facility protocol/manufacturer guidelines when encountering portable VADs.

HeartMate LVADs are small, sturdy, quiet, and implantable, and several versions exist. They are frequently used as a bridge to transplant. However, their use is also considered a destination therapy because of their ability to provide long-term, mechanical circulatory support to patients with heart failure without the expectation of a transplant.

A pulsitile, or rotary pump, is implanted into the abdomen and attached to the heart. The pump is controlled by a small external monitor that the patient can carry in a pack around the waist for up to 8 hours. This allows freedom of movement.

The portable monitor is attached to a power base (which houses a system controller) when the patient is at home, where it is recharged. The HeartMate can produce a blood flow rate as high as 10 L per minute. Its portability allows a patient to go home, go to work, and resume normal activities.

The Thoratec IVAD is used for right, left, or biventricular function as a bridge to transplant. Its pump can be internal or external. A patient can go home with either type of pump because they both use a portable compressor system about the size of backpack.

Other VADs exist but are not as commonplace as the devices discussed above. However, their function and support may be as great—or even exceed—those mentioned.

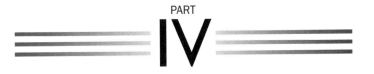

PART

IV

The Specialty Critical Care Unit

14

Surgical and Orthopedic Recovery Guidelines

INTRODUCTION

Surgical and orthopedic patients generally recover in the post-anesthesia care unit. They are transferred to the nursing floor, after meeting certain parameters, and discharged when appropriate. However, there are times when this group requires specialized nursing care and additional medical support.

Chest-tube management, wound care, central venous pressure (CVP) monitoring, pain management, and the prevention of pulmonary problems and deep vein thrombus (DVT) are important aspects of nursing implementation when providing post-surgical care.

Orthopedic surgery is extremely common, with some patients requiring ICU support. Proper turning and positioning, as well as care techniques for those in traction or external fixation, are valuable skills used in the critical care environment.

In this chapter you will learn:

1. Proper chest-tube set-up, management, and removal techniques.
2. The ins and outs of CVP monitoring.
3. Wound care guidelines for post-surgical patients.
4. Guidelines for the care of post-operative orthopedic patients.
5. Tips for preventing post-surgical pulmonary problems and DVT.

CHEST TUBES

A chest tube (CT) is inserted for a variety of reasons, such as empyema, hemothorax, pleural effusion, and pneumothorax. **Its primary function is to drain air, blood, and/ or fluid from the pleural space, giving the lungs a chance to re-expand.** It also re-establishes negative pressure. A CT is inserted, using aseptic technique, by an advanced practioner, and placement is confirmed with a chest x-ray. **The type of tube discussed in this chapter is inserted into the pleural space.** However, mediastinal CTs and drains are inserted post-coronary artery bypass graft (CABG) surgery to prevent fluid buildup around the heart. These are further explained in Chapter 16.

CTs are connected to a drainage system composed of two parts: a collection container and a seal that stops air from entering the chest when the patient breathes. Most drainage systems work on a three-bottle system consisting of a drainage compartment, a water-seal compartment, and a final compartment that is connected to suction and controls pressure.

In most facilities, a Pleur-evac unit is used and houses the three compartments. The first collects drainage from the patient via a tube connected to the actual CT. The second is the water-seal and contains approximately 2 cm of H_2O. It provides the seal. The third provides suction. The amount of suction is determined by the amount of H_2O in the compartment. Usually, the prescribed or manufacturer-recommended level is –20 cm H_2O.

FAST FACTS in a NUTSHELL

To set up a Pleur-evac 3-compartment unit:

1. Stand the unit on the floor or counter-top to prepare.
2. Using the funnel provided or a 50-ml syringe, fill the water-seal compartment with sterile water or normal saline to the 2-cm mark.
3. Fill the suction control compartment with the same solution to the ordered level.
4. Connect the tubing from the suction control compartment to suction mode.
5. Connect the tubing from the drainage compartment to the CT or leave the sterile cover in place to maintain sterility until the CT is inserted.

(Adapted from Alspach, 2006; Chohan & Munden, 2007; Ehlers, 2007; Nettina, 2010; Wyckoff et al., 2009.)

For the preparation of other types of CT drainage systems, refer to manufacturer/facility policies and procedures.

Tidaling should be observed in the water-seal chamber. The fluid level should get higher upon inspiration and lower upon exhalation during spontaneous respirations. If a ventilator is being used, the opposite should occur. This oscillation will not occur if the lung has re-expanded or the tubing is blocked. If no fluid variation is noted, encourage coughing and deep breathing, if applicable, and/or reposition the patient. If there is no change, notify the physician.

A small amount of intermittent bubbling should be observed in the water-seal. However, large or new bubbling can signify an air leak. Check all connections and assess for cracks or holes in the drainage system. Notify the physician if the new bubbling persists.

For a drainage system not employing water, the negative pressure and suction gauges should be closely monitored to prevent too much negative pressure.

==*FAST FACTS in a NUTSHELL*

Complications of CT placement and therapy include bleeding, hemothorax, infection, intercostal artery tear, pain, perforation of visceral organs, subcutaneous emphysema, and tube occlusion.

Guidelines to follow when assisting with the insertion of a CT:

- Confirm consent and patient identity via two patient identifiers.
- Educate the patient and family, and provide emotional support.
- Pre-medicate the patient, as ordered.
- Set up CT drainage system prior to tube insertion.
- CT size varies from 18 to 40 French. Ask the advanced practioner which tube is needed or have a variety available.
- Position the patient supine, on the edge of the bed, with the opposite arm raised above the head, if possible. Otherwise, place a rolled towel behind the shoulder to open up the intercostal space.
- A CT insertion kit may be available. If not, have the following, sterile, at the bedside:
    1. Chest tube
    2. 1% lidocaine
    3. 21-, 22-, and 25-gauge needles
    4. Several syringes, in varying sizes
    5. Kelly clamps × 2
    6. #11 surgical blade/knife
    7. Appropriate PPE
    8. 0-silk suture
    9. Drain sponges, gauze, and 4×4s
    10. Petroleum gauze
- Have tape at bedside.
- CTs are generally inserted above the sixth intercostal space.
- Prepare insertion site using aseptic technique.

- Prepare sterile field and drape patient.
- Monitor vital signs (VS) and respiratory status closely during CT insertion.
- After insertion, confirm that a chest x-ray has been taken and read.
- Document the procedure, patient tolerance, and drainage characteristics.

Nursing implementations involved in the care of a patient with a CT include:

- Monitor vital signs and O_2 saturation frequently.
- Assess respirations, observing:
  1. Rate
  2. Rhythm
  3. Breath sounds
  4. Subcutaneous emphysema
- Assess type, color, and amount of CT drainage.
- Always maintain the drainage system below the chest level of the patient.
- Check tubing for kinks or blockages.
- Do not allow dependent loops in tubing.
- Secure tubing connections with tape.
- Mark drainage level with date and time on the drainage unit.
- Call MD for CT drainage >200 ml in 1 hour.
- Call MD if no CT drainage is noted.
- Call MD for changes in respiratory status.
- Call MD stat for deviated trachea.
- Medicate for pain, as ordered.
- Inspect insertion site frequently for bleeding, drainage, and odor.
- Change dressing daily and PRN, using aseptic technique.
- Maintain suction at manufacturer-suggested or MD-prescribed amount.
- Add H_2O to water-seal compartment PRN.
- Do not clamp a CT if the patient has had a thoracotomy or has a tracheobronchial leak.

- If any other CT must be clamped (e.g., to change the drainage system), do not forget to unclamp prior to the 1-minute mark.
- If patient transport is required, do not clamp the tubing. Remove the tubing from the suction port. The drainage system will continue to function even when not attached to suction via venting.
- Do not milk or strip a CT.
- Confirm that a daily chest x-ray is taken and read.
- If a CT is inadvertently removed, cover the site with petroleum gauze. Notify MD stat. Assess respiratory status. Place a three-sided taped dressing to the site that will allow air to escape on exhalation. This may help prevent a tension pneumothorax.
- Perform range-of-motion (ROM) exercises, as tolerated.
- Turn patient at least every 2 hours if not contraindicated.
- Encourage coughing and deep breathing, if possible.

(Adapted from Alspach, 2006; Chohan & Munden, 2007; Ehlers, 2007; Nettina, 2010; Stillwell, 2006; Wyckoff et al., 2009.)

CT removal is performed at the bedside once it has been determined that all drainage and air leaks have been resolved. Temporary clamping may be initiated prior to removal to confirm resolution of the medical issue and observe patient tolerance.

An advanced practioner needs certain supplies, such as a suture removal kit, petroleum gauze, sterile 4 × 4s, and tape, at the bedside to remove a CT. **Pre-medicate the patient, as ordered.** The CT will be removed in one swift movement while the patient practices the Valsalva maneuver. After a dressing is applied, a chest x-ray should be taken to evaluate reaccumulation of fluid or return of pneumothorax or hemothorax. Frequent and accurate assessments of respiratory status must follow CT removal.

CENTRAL VENOUS PRESSURE MONITORING

Central venous pressure (**CVP) monitoring is performed to assess the function of the heart and evaluate fluid status. It is equal to the pressure of the right atrium (RA).**

A CVP catheter is inserted into a large vein such as the femoral, jugular, median basilic, or subclavian. **The tip rests in the superior vena cava,** about 2 cm above the RA. The line may be single-lumen, just for reading CVP, or have multiple lumens that can be used to monitor CVP, draw blood, and administer fluid and medications.

The insertion process, care, and removal of a CVP catheter are similar to those for a central venous line. Refer to Chapter 9 for guidelines. Ensure that the CVP transducer has been zeroed prior to insertion. **A small waveform, normally ranging from 2 to 6 mmHg,** will be noted on the monitor when the catheter is properly connected and transduced. This pressure is read in mean and monitored continuously.

════════════════════════════════*FAST FACTS in a NUTSHELL*

Complications of CVP catheter insertion and monitoring include: air embolus, pericardial effusion, cardiac tamponade, catherter migration, hemorrhage, hemothorax, infection, pneumothorax, thrombus, ventricular dysrhythmias, and vessel damage.

A few tips pertaining to CVP monitoring follow:

- If a tall waveform with pressures ranging from 25 to 30 mmHg is noted, suspect catheter migration into the right ventricle (RV). Notify the MD stat.
- Continuously monitor the EKG.
- Ensure that monitor alarm parameters are correct for the patient and on.
- For a change in CVP reading of greater than 2, notify MD.
- Maintain the transducer level with the phlebostatic axis.
- Relevel and zero the transducer with patient re-positioning.
- Read pressure waveform at end-expiration.
- Confirm that a chest x-ray is taken daily.
- Frequently assess respiratory status.
- Troubleshooting tips for CVP pressure monitoring are similar to those for a PA catheter. Refer to Chapter 11.

(Adapted from Alspach, 2006; Chohan & Munden, 2007; Ehlers, 2007; Nettina, 2010; Stillwell, 2006; Wyckoff et al., 2009.)

POST-SURGICAL WOUND CARE

Surgical wound care is performed to prevent infection and help a wound heal properly. The following guidelines for post-op incision and wound care are general, as actual physician's orders vary:

- Dry dressings are used for wounds closed by primary intention.
- Wet-to-dry dressings are used to close wounds by secondary intention. These sites are often contaminated.
- Wet-to-wet dressing are used on clean, open sites or granulations.
- Pouching (completed to appear almost like an ostomy bag) can be applied to protect the surrounding skin from corrosive drainage.
- Complete dressing changes as ordered and PRN to keep the site dry.
- Try not to perform dressing changes around mealtime.
- Certain MDs want to perform the first post-op dressing change.Verify this information prior to removing the initial dressing.
- Confirm patient identity via two identifiers.
- Verify any patient allergies.
- Provide patient/family education and emotional support.
- Pre-medicate the patient, as ordered, prior to removing old dressing.
- Evaluate lab work, such as the white blood cell count.
- Note VS, particularly temperature.
- Gather needed supplies prior to entering the patient's room.
- Use aseptic technique.
- Document the appearance and odor of drainage on old dressings.
- Assess wound for approximation, redness, dehiscence, and evisceration.
- Assess the appearance of sutures, staples, and/or steri-strips.

- Do not use cotton balls.
- Obtain a culture, if applicable, prior to cleaning the wound.
- Clean the incision/wound with sterile saline.
- Never apply povidone-iodine or chlorhexidine directly to a surgical site.
- For two sites in the same vicinity, cleanse and dress each separately.
- Clean the site properly. The incision line is cleaner than the surrounding skin; the top of the line (if vertical) is considered cleaner than the bottom.
- Clean 1 inch beyond the dressing site. If no further dressing changes are required, clean 2 inches beyond the dressing site.
- If a drain is in place, clean it last, working from the drain insertion site outward.
- Maintain drain tubing away from incision site.
- Irrigate the site, if ordered.
- Administer topical medication, if ordered.
- Pack wound, if ordered.
- Do not pack wound extremely tight.
- A T-binder or Montgomery straps may be used for dressings requiring frequent changes.
- Using a skin-prep solution on surrounding skin may help tape adhere and minimize skin irritation.
- A skin protectant cream/lotion can be applied to surrounding skin to help reduce irritation from excoriating drainage, such as that of the GI tract.
- Use a drain sponge, if applicable. If none is available, use two-folded, non-cotton-lined gauze pads with slits cut into them to surround drain tubing.
- Use a surgical mask to support (it supports a dressimg, not replaces it) a chin or jaw dressing.
- The most drainage generally occurs during the first 24 hours post-op.
- Empty drains at least once a shift, as ordered, and PRN. Document appearance, amount, and odor of drainage.

(Adapted from Alexander, 2006; Ehlers, 2007; Foreman et al., 2010; Nettina, 2010.)

POST-SURGICAL ORTHOPEDIC CARE

For patients recovering from orthopedic surgery, frequent assessment of peripheral pulses, sensation, color, temperature, and capillary refill is needed. Immobilization of the op-site extremity is necessary and activity is limited, according to the type of surgery performed. Patients are closely monitored for hemorrhage and shock related to the knowledge that orthopedic surgical incisions tend to bleed more than those of other surgeries, particularly in the first 24 hours. Pain management is of the utmost importance.

The ICU often has total hip-replacement patients, and certain positioning techniques are needed when providing post-op care. Supine is the most common patient position. The operative hip is placed in minimal abduction via a splint, pillow, or Buck's traction. It should not be adducted or flexed. The head of the bed should be no greater than 45° to 60°. Two caregivers must be available when turning the patient to provide adequate support to the operative hip and leg.

════════════════════════════*FAST FACTS in a NUTSHELL*

Complications arising from orthopedic surgery include anemia, atelectasis, compartment syndrome, pulmonary embolus, bleeding, infection, and pneumonia.

TRACTION

Traction is required following some types of orthopedic surgery. It is applied to either the skin or skeleton. Several steps need to be taken in the care of patients in traction:

- Provide patient/family education and emotional support.
- Obtain an orthopedic bed with a traction frame.
- Obtain needed weights, rope, or pulleys.

- Clean pin sites with facility-approved solution. Biopatch may be ordered.
- Follow advanced practioner instructions regarding traction application.
- Maintain patient's head neutrally when positioning traction.
- Allow weights to hang freely.
- Do not allow a knot in the rope near a pulley.
- Do not allow ropes to touch the bed or any equipment.
- Do not allow the footplate to touch the pulley or the foot of the bed.
- Confirm that the pull is in line with the long axis of the bone.
- Keep patient body alignment neutral: in line with pulleys and ropes.
- Turn the patient every 2 hours and PRN, if not contraindicated.
- Do not remove the weights of skeletal traction when turning or moving a patient.
- Logroll the patient when turning; provide adequate support to maintain alignment.
- Assess skin thoroughly, including surgical and pin sites.
- Monitor VS and temperature.
- Assess the treated extremity frequently.
- Palpate peripheral pulses often.
- Provide adequate pain relief.
- Place pin coverings over sharp ends of skeletal traction.
- Maintain wrinkle-free linens & gown.
- Use heel and elbow protectors.

(Adapted from Ehlers, 2007; Nettina, 2010.)

═══════════════════════════*FAST FACTS in a NUTSHELL*

Complications from traction include infection, loss of sensation, muscle spasms, numbness, pain, and skin breakdown.

EXTERNAL FIXATION

External fixation involves inserting pins through the skin and bone and attaching the pins to an external metal frame. This is often used to stabilize open fractures with extreme soft-tissue injury and is applied in the OR. The physician generally completes post-application adjustments. Complications of external fixation are similar to those of traction.

Care guidelines for patients with external fixation:

- Cover sharp, exposed pin ends.
- Provide patient/family education and emotional support.
- Assess pulse, sensation, color, temperature, and capillary refill of extremity undergoing treatment.
- Assess pin sites and any wounds for redness, swelling, pain, and drainage.
- Provide adequate pain management.
- Turn patient every 2 hours and PRN, if possible.
- Clean pin sites and wound per facility protocol.
- Clean fixator with water, PRN.
- Elevate extremity, PRN.

(Adapted from Ehlers, 2007; Nettina, 2010.)

PREVENTING POST-OP PULMONARY PROBLEMS AND DEEP VEIN THROMBOSIS PROPHYLAXIS

Pulmonary Problems

═══════════════════════*FAST FACTS in a NUTSHELL*

Post-op surgical patients are at increased risk for development of pulmonary issues, such as aspiration, atelectasis, microatelectasis, and pneumonia. These complications lead to poor healing, longer hospital stays, increased medical costs, and increased patient morbidity.

To help prevent post-op problems, multiple nursing implementations can be completed:

- Educate patient/family and provide emotional support.
- Provide adequate pain management.
- Perform and encourage oral hygiene.
- Elevate HOB, as tolerated.
- Administer oxygen therapy, as ordered.
- Encourage coughing and deep breathing, along with incisional splinting, every 2 hours, if possible.
- Suction PRN.
- Observe sputum/secretions for changes in color, texture, odor, and amount.
- Encourage use of incentive spirometry every 2 hours, if applicable.
- Closely monitor respiratory status and breath sounds.
- Monitor O_2 saturation.
- Check VS, temperature, and hemodynamics frequently.
- Assess nail beds for changes in color.
- Reposition the patient; turn every 2 hours.
- Perform ROM, if possible. Consult physical therapist, per protocol.
- Ambulate early, if not contraindicated.

DEEP VEIN THROMBOSIS PROPHYLAXIS

The development of a deep vein thrombosis (DVT) is as high as 40% in the post-surgical hospital population (Nettina, 2010). These Thrombi have the potential to become dangerous pulmonary emboli, causing major complications.

═══════════════════════════════════════*FAST FACTS in a NUTSHELL*

DVTs often have no signs or symptoms. However, some observations to note include pain or cramping in the calf or thigh, a minimal fever with or without chills and sweating, and changes in the pedal pulses or size of limbs.

DVT prophylaxis is usually a standard post-op protocol. Orders and implementations vary among facilities, surgery types, and practioners. General guidelines for the prevention of DVT follow:

- Provide patient/family education and emotional support.
- Frequently assess capillary refill, peripheral pulses, and thigh/calf/foot sensation/ and girth.
- Administer anticoagulation, as ordered.
- Provide adequate hydration.
- Test for positive Homan's sign.
- Do not massage calf/thigh.
- Turn the patient every 2 hours, if possible.
- Do not place rolls behind the patient's knees.
- Perform ROM, if not contraindicated.
- Use sequential compression devices and foot pumps, as ordered.
- Ambulate early, if possible.

(Adapted from Nettina, 2010; Stillwell, 2006.)

15

The Neuro ICU

INTRODUCTION

Every critical care unit encounters patients with changing dynamics who require constant monitoring, skilled care, and nurses who love their specialty. The neurological intensive care unit (NICU) is no exception. Its population suffers from diagnoses such as cranial aneurysms, encephalopathy, head trauma, increased intracranial pressure (ICP), seizures, stroke, and spinal cord injuries.

Such intricate issues necessitate specialized interventions, devices, and treatment. The Glasgow Coma Scale (GCS) and additional strategies are employed to complete comprehensive neurological assessments. Monitoring devices used in the NICU include jugular venous oxygen saturation ($SjvO_2$), transcranial Doppler (TCD), and electroencephalogram (EEG).

In this chapter you will learn:

1. The specifics of the GCS and guidelines for a complete neurological assessment.
2. ICP management, including how to care for and troubleshoot a ventricular catheter.

3. Strategies involved in the insertion and troubleshooting of an SjvO₂ catheter.
4. The definition of a TCD and EEG.

NEUROLOGICAL ASSESSMENT

Completion of a comprehensive neurological assessment is an important aspect of caring for a patient in the NICU. The basics of such an assessment are detailed in Chapter 5, Figure 5.1, along with guidelines for performing a physical assessment. The entire physical assessment is performed because several portions are needed to acquire an overall picture of a patient's neurological function and/or deficits. In addition, several other evaluation techniques should be employed, if applicable, during a complete neurological examination:

1. Level of consciousness
2. GCS; see Figure 15.1
3. Observe for papilledema
4. Motor function
5. Sensory function
6. Eye movements; gaze
7. Pain; headache
8. Nausea/vomiting
9. Cranial nerves
10. Strength testing
11. Muscle tone
12. Deep tendon reflexes
13. Superficial reflexes

(Adapted from Alspach, 2006; Chohan & Munden, 2007; Nettina, 2010; Stillwell, 2006; Wyckoff et al., 2009.)

Physicians and other members of the health care team use these components to determine a baseline for a patient that acts as a scale to evaluate medical, physical, and neurological status.

Numerous tests can uncover the cause of changes in neurological function and assist with determining the course of treatment. ABGs, blood work, cerebral angiography,

Figure 15.1 The Glasgow Coma Scale

Response	Score
Eye Opening:	
• Spontaneous: blinks/opens eyes without stimulation	4
• To verbal stimulus or command	3
• To pain only	2
• No response to stimulus	1
Verbal Response:	
• Oriented	5
• Confused, but answers questions	4
• Inappropriate words	3
• Incomprehensible sounds	2
• None (A "T" may be noted to acknowledge trach/ETT)	1
Motor Response:	
• Obeys/follows commands	6
• Localizes: tries to remove stimulus	5
• Withdraws from stimulus	4
• Abnormal flexion, decorticate posturing	3
• Abnormal extension, decerebrate posturing	2
• No movement in response to stimulus	1

Note: A score of 15 is considered normal.

(Adapted from Alspach, 2006; Centers for Disease Control and Prevention, 2010; Nettina, 2010; Rowlett, 2000; Wyckoff et al., 2009.)

cerebrospinal fluid (CSF) analysis, CT scan, EEG, evoked potentials, lumbar puncture, nerve conduction studies, magnetic resonance angiography (MRA), magnetic resonance imaging (MRI), myelography, positron emission tomography (PET), single photon emission tomography (SPECT), spinal angiography, toxicology screens, transcranial Doppler, urinalysis, and x-rays are all options used to diagnose under-lying pathologies and conditions.

INTRACRANIAL PRESSURE (ICP) MANAGEMENT

ICP is the measurement of the pressure that blood, CSF, and the brain itself place on the skull. The normal range for an adult is 5–15 mmHg. Increased ICP is an emergency situation that requires immediate treatment to prevent brain ischemia. It is a frequent complication of neurological issues, such as intracranial hemorrhage, cerebral edema, traumatic brain injury, brain tumors, problems involving CSF, seizures, and stroke. **There are four basic types of ICP monitoring**: an epidural sensor, intraparenchymal pressure monitor, subarachnoid bolt, and ventricular catheter. The ventricular catheter is the most commonly used.

VENTRICULAR CATHETER

A ventricular, or intraventricular catheter is inserted into the non-dominant ventricle of the brain via a burr hole drilled into the skull. This procedure is completed either in the OR or at the bedside using aseptic technique. The patient is placed supine and the head of the bed is positioned at an angle of 30–45 degrees.

This type of device is generally considered the most accurate way to measure ICP. It is also an important tool for ICP management, as CSF can be drained by the catheter. Ventriculostomies and external ventricular drains (EVDs) are both ventricular catheters.

The catheter is attached to an external, preservative-free, saline-filled system that is capable of drainage. The pressure measurement is transduced, using the top of the external auditory canal (foramen of Monro) as a reference point for leveling, unless otherwise specified by the physician. It will drain when the CSF drainage system is connected distal to the external transducer.

The readings displayed on the monitor are continuous and accurate when the device is properly calibrated and leveled. Frequent recalibrations are required during therapy. **Alarms should be on and set according to patient status.** No constant flush is used with ICP monitoring, as it could increase ICP.

The ventricular catheter site is kept clean and dry with an occlusive dressing. **Aseptic technique is imperative when working with a ventricular catheter.**

FAST FACTS in a NUTSHELL

The completion of an ICP reading from a ventricular catheter is fairly easy:

1. Zero and relevel the transducer with the external auditory canal, or as ordered.
2. Close the CSF drainage system, if applicable.
3. Perform an ICP reading at end-expiration.

(Adapted from Ehlers, 2007; Kirchman, 2010; Nettina, 2010; Stillwell, 2006; Wyckoff et al., 2009.)

ICP readings are displayed on the monitor connected to the transducer and system. The waveform closely mimics the appearance of a CVP tracing. **The waveform is small and monitored in mean.** It normally has three peaks; however, more may be observed for certain patients.

Troubleshooting tips for the ventricular catheter:

- Confirm proper zero procedure with manufacturer guidelines and/or facility policy.
- Re-level the transducer with the external auditory meatus upon patient position changes and any handling of the system.
- Confirm that no air is in the saline-filled system.
- Catheter may only be flushed if specifically ordered by the physician.
- *Dampened waveform:* Indicative of possible catheter obstruction, air in the system, or loose system

connections. Attempt to remove air from line. Flush the system, not the catheter. Do not push air towards the patient. Check and tighten system connections. Notify the physician if problem persists.

- *False high or low-pressure reading:* Re-level the transducer. Check for air in line and remove, if possible.
- Notify the physician stat for a high ICP reading, lasting more than 1–2 minutes.
- During patient transport, maintain proper transducer level or turn the drainage off until patient is moved and re-settled.
- Notify the physician if there is no CSF drainage, too much CSF drainage, or if changes in CSF appearance are noted.

(Adapted from Alspach, 2006; Chohan & Munden, 2007; Ehlers, 2007; Kirchman, 2010; Nettina, 2010; Stillwell, 2006.)

═══════════════*FAST FACTS in a NUTSHELL*

CSF drains by gravity and can be constant or intermittent, per physician parameters. Some guidelines regarding the CSF drainage system:

- The drip chamber can be attached to the headboard or an IV pole at the bedside.
- Level the air-fluid interface with the foramen of Monroe, or as ordered.
- Ensure that the drip chamber is not too high or too low; both could cause changes to CSF drainage and/or ICP.
- Document CSF drainage amount and appearance, hourly and PRN.
- The CSF drainage system is sterile. If a bag change is required, practice aseptic technique. Label the new drainage bag with date, time, and initials.

(Adapted from Alspach, 2006; Chohan & Munden, 2007; Ehlers, 2007; Kirchman, 2010; Nettina, 2010; Stillwell, 2006.)

A physician's order is needed to obtain a CSF sample for analysis. It is performed using aseptic technique. Follow facility-specific protocol for sample attainment, noting the amount of CSF required for the tests ordered.

A physician, using aseptic technique, removes the ventricular catheter. The site is covered with a sterile dressing for a minimum of 24 hours. It is then left open to air.

═══════════════════════════════*FAST FACTS in a NUTSHELL*

Complications involved with ventricular catheter use include infection, catheter obstruction, hemorrhage, brain ischemia, and death. Contraindications to most types of ICP monitoring are stenotic cerebral ventricles and vascular lesions.

OTHER TYPES OF ICP MONITORING

A subarachnoid bolt (SAB) is a fluid-filled system that monitors ICP. It is inserted via a burr hole. A bolt, prepped with preservative-free saline, is inserted and contacts the subarachnoid space. ICP is then transduced through the system.

This device is easily inserted at the bedside and has a lower risk of infection than a ventricular catheter. However, the SAB frequently becomes obstructed, is not capable of CSF drainage, requires frequent re-calibration, and is considered less accurate than a ventricular catheter.

An epidural catheter is placed, via a small drill hole, with its catheter tip resting in the epidural space. It is less invasive than both a ventricular catheter and SAB, easy to insert, does not require re-calibration, and has a low infection rate. However, epidural catheters often break down, do not allow for CSF drainage, are inaccurate, and can become dislocated.

An intraparenchymal pressure monitor is a fiber-optic, transducer-tipped catheter that is inserted via a bolt into the ventricle, subdural space, or intraparenchymal tissue. It is easy to insert, exhibits adequate readings, and requires only one calibration, which is completed upon insertion. However, it does not provide for CSF drainage and quickly breaks.

ADDITIONAL ICP MANAGEMENT

Several things have the potential to increase ICP, such as extreme head, neck, or hip flexion, fluid overload, head rotation >90 degrees, hypercapnia, hypoxia, REM sleep, suctioning, the Valsalva maneuver, and inadequate rest between activities.

Completing various **medical treatments, administering medications, and performing certain nursing implementations** reduce the risk of increased ICP. Examples of some interventions include:

- Maintain the head of the bed at 30 degrees, unless contraindicated.
- Maintain neck in the neutral position.
- Prevent hypothermia/hyperthermia.
- Do not rapidly re-warm or cool the patient.
- Prevent shivering, if possible.
- Closely monitor neurological status, VS, hemodynamics, and respirations.
- Maintain $PaCO_2$ at 35–45 mmHg.
- Maintain PEEP <10 cm H_2O, if applicable.
- Suction only when absolutely necessary.
- Maintain BP, per physician parameters.
- Monitor fluid status closely and adjust PRN. Fluid restriction is often ordered.
- Maintain blood glucose within normal limits, as ordered.

- Monitor for seizures and control, as ordered.
- Manage pain adequately.
- Treat/prevent agitation, PRN, as ordered.
- Administration of mannitol (Osmitol, Resectisol) to decrease cerebral edema:
    1. Assess electrolyte levels and osmolality prior to administration.
    2. If ordered, give 50 cc 5% albumin with mannitol to reduce rebound increased ICP.
- Administration of loop diuretics, such as furosemide (Lasix).
- Glucocorticoid administration
- Lidocaine administration
- Administration of hypertonic saline (2% or 3%).
- Induction of a "medication" coma to reduce the metabolic demand of the brain.
- Controlled hyperventilation
- Insertion of a nasogastric tube and/or urinary catheter.
- Reversal/improvement of the underlying condition/pathology causing increased ICP.
- Educate the patient and family regarding:
    1. Patient status
    2. Procedures
    3. Proper body alignment importance
    4. Restriction of the Valsalva maneuver
- Provide a calm, quiet environment.

(Adapted from Alspach, 2006; Chohan & Munden, 2007; Ehlers, 2007; Kirchman, 2010; Nettina, 2010; Stillwell, 2006, Wyckoff et al., 2009.)

JUGULAR VENOUS OXYGEN SATURATION

Jugular venous oximetry measures jugular venous oxygen saturation ($SjvO_2$). A fiber-optic, oximetric catheter is inserted into an introducer, similar to a CVL, using sterile technique. The tip rests in the jugular bulb of the internal jugular vein and is connected to a monitor.

The reading is the oxygen saturation of the blood after cerebral perfusion has occurred. **Normal SjvO$_2$ is 55–75 %.** A high reading is indicative of brain hyperperfusion. A low reading is indicative of brain ischemia and/or increased ICP. ICP and SjvO$_2$ are often monitored simultaneously.

To assist with the insertion of an SjvO$_2$ catheter, the following guidelines are used:

- Confirm the patient's identity via 2 patient identifiers.
- Provide patient/family education.
- Gather the required supplies and equipment.
- Put on sterile gloves.
- Prime the pressure tubing and calibrate the system per manufacturer/facility protocol.
- Position the patient with the neck neutral.
- Elevate the head of the bed 30–45 degrees.
- Prep the patient and sterile field in a similar fashion to a central line insertion, per facility protocol. Refer to Chapter 9 for details.
- Ensure that a 5 Fr introducer and 4 Fr SjvO$_2$ catheter are at the bedside.
- Assist the physician with donning of PPE.
- Monitor patient closely during catheter insertion by the physician.
- Connect the pressure tubing.
- Aspirate blood and flush both jugular catheter lumens.
- Clean site.
- Apply sterile, occlusive dressing.
- Aspirate a blood sample for a jugular blood gas analysis.
- Document SjvO$_2$ reading and patient tolerance of the procedure.
- Confirm that a chest x-ray is taken and read.

(Adapted from Alspach, 2006; Chohan & Munden, 2007; Ehlers, 2007; Nettina, 2010.)

===============*FAST FACTS in a NUTSHELL*

Tips for troubleshooting an $SjvO_2$ reading:

- Confirm the accuracy of the reading by drawing an $SjvO_2$ blood gas every 8 hours. If the reading is within 4% of the analysis, it is considered accurate.
- Calibrate the system each shift, per manufacturer guidelines.
- Aspirate blood slowly, approximately 1 ml/min.
- *Low light intensity:* Notify the physician; anticipate catheter replacement.
- *High light intensity:* Position patient's head to neutral; possible vessel artifact.
- *Catheter occlusion:* Aspirate blood until it is freely withdrawn and normal light intensity is noted.
- Rhythmic changes in the reading are indicative of catheter coiling. Notify the physician. Anticipate a chest x-ray and possible catheter replacement.
- For sustained elevated ICP of more than 5 mmHg over patient baseline post-$SjvO_2$ catheter insertion, anticipate removal of $SjvO_2$ catheter.
- Notify the physician of desaturations.

(Adapted from Alspach, 2006; Chohan & Munden, 2007; Ehlers, 2007; Nettina, 2010.)

$SjvO_2$ **catheters are removed similar to central venous lines and PA catheters.** Refer to Chapters 9 and 11 for the steps. The complications related to $SjvO_2$ catheter insertion and monitoring are bleeding, carotid artery puncture, impaired venous drainage, increased ICP, pneumothorax, and thrombus.

OTHER NEUROLOGICAL MONITORING MODALITIES

Transcranial Doppler (TCD) is a type of ultrasonography used to determine if there are blockages in the vessels that provide blood flow to the brain. It can also detect vasospasm. This modality is non-invasive, provides immediate results, is performed at the bedside, and is absolutely painless.

An **EEG is used to measure electrical activity in the brain.** Electrodes are attached to the scalp. Continuous EEG monitoring can be performed at the bedside. It is helpful in diagnosing seizures and capable of observing areas of brain ischemia. It is painless and noninvasive.

16

General Cardiac Care and Post-Coronary-Artery-Bypass-Graft Patients

INTRODUCTION

According to the American Heart Association, over 81,000,000 people in the United States were known to have cardiovascular disease in 2006. Approximately 830,000 of those died from complications caused by the disease.

Considering that, of the survivors, almost 18 million have already had an acute myocardial infarction or an episode of angina, it is extremely important that every critical care nurse be skilled in the interventions these patients require. ICU nurses frequently encounter patients with cardiac problems, even if they work in a non-cardiac unit.

In this chapter you will learn:

1. General cardiac care guidelines.
2. How to prepare and help a patient recover from cardiac catheterization and/or an electrophysiology study.

3. Proper aterial and venous sheath removal techniques.
4. Recovery guidelines for post-coronary-artery-bypass-graft patients.

CARDIAC CARE

Patients in the ICU often require cardiac care, even if it is not the primary reason for their hospital admission. Basic implementations for providing cardiac care follow:

- Compile a complete medical history with details pertaining to current medical complaints (e.g., chest pain/shortness of breath onset and exacerbating factors), cardiac history, family cardiac history, current medications, allergies, etc.
- Perform a complete physical assessment (refer to Chapter 5). Apply specific attention to pulses, neck veins, heart sounds (noting any murmurs), and breath sounds.
- Monitor VS and hemodynamics.
- Monitor EKG; see Appendix B for basic rhythm strip interpretation.
- Complete a 12 lead EKG; see Appendix C for lead placement.
- Assess lab results; particularly blood glucose (BG), brain natriuretic peptide (BNP), CBC, clotting factors, creatinine kinase (CK), C-reactive protein, electrolytes, myoglobin, troponin I, and troponin T.
- Confirm completion of diagnostic tests such as a chest x-ray, CT, MRI, and stress test.
- Notify MD of lab results, test results, new patient complaints, and changes in VS, hemodynamics, and/or assessment.
- Administer medications, such as amiodarone (Cordarone), nitroglycerin, heparin, clopidogrel (Plavix), statins, etc., as ordered.
- Maintain IV & CVL sites, per protocol. See Chapter 9 for care details.

- Titrate vasoactive drips, such as dopamine, dobutamine (Dobutrex), epinephrine, norepinephrine (Levophed), and nitroglycerin, to maintain VS and hemodynamics within ordered parameters.
- Turn the patient every 2 hours.
- Provide adequate skin and oral care.
- Provide adequate nutritional intake.
- Consult nutritionists, dieticians, physical therapists, occupational therapists, and other members of the health care team PRN.
- Provide patient/family education and emotional support.

A team approach to cardiac care improves patient outcomes. It is extremely important to involve the patient and family members.

CARDIAC CATHETERIZATION

A cardiac catheterization is completed in the cardiac catheterization lab (CCL). A cardiologist, using sterile technique, performs the procedure. **During a left-sided heart catheterization, the femoral artery, usually the right, is accessed via a sheath.** Occasionally a brachial artery is accessed. The radial artery is rarely used. Catheters are inserted into the openings of the coronary arteries, guided by fluoroscopy. Contrast is injected to visualize the coronaries. Any abnormalities and/or blockages, are noted. The cardiac anatomy, valves, and function are observed. **Angioplasty, stent placement, and/or atherectomy are performed,** as determined by the physician.

During a right-sided heart catheterization, pulmonary artery pressures are assessed and a cardiac tissue biopsy can be obtained. This is done via an antecubital or femoral vein. The catheters are also guided by fluoroscopy.

The patient is sedated during these procedures for pain relief and anxiety reduction. **Moderate "conscious" sedation is generally administered.** However, general anesthesia is sometimes required.

===============*FAST FACTS in a NUTSHELL*

Medications that may be administered are heparin, bivalirudin (Angiomax), clopidogrel (Plavix), a glycoprotein IIb IIIa inhibitor, aspirin, and/or vasoactive drips. **Some medications may be continued in the ICU.**

Guidelines for preparation for a cardiac catheterization include:

1. Confirm the MD order.
2. Verify the patient's identity via two facility-approved identifiers.
3. Confirm consent.
4. Provide patient/family education and emotional support.
5. Verify patient allergies. Be alert to contrast, shellfish, and iodine sensitivity; if encountered, notify MD.
6. Confirm patient medications and any held the day of the procedure. Warfarin (Coumadin) is frequently held 3 days prior to the procedure. Medications containing metformin (Glucophage) should be the held the day of the test.
7. Pre-medicate, as ordered.
8. Follow facility policy regarding NPO status; usually 4 to 6 hours NPO prior to initiation of the procedure.
9. Ensure patent IV.
10. Assess BUN/creatinine, CBC, electrolytes, and WBC. Notify MD of abnormalities.
11. Assess and mark pedal and post-tibial pulses.
12. Clip hair at access site. Follow facility protocol for cleansing.

At most facilities, the cardiac catheterization team has patients recover in a holding room. At others, patients report directly back to the ICU. Either way, the steps of recovery are similar:

1. Assess VS and hemodynamics every 15 minutes ×4 and every 30 minutes ×4, followed by routine assessment, if the patient is stable.
2. Continuously monitor EKG.
3. Maintain oxygen saturation >92%, applying supplemental oxygen PRN.
4. Assess access site with each VS check: treat changes per protocol.
5. Assess pain at least hourly ×12 hours.
6. Assess peripheral pulses, applicable to access site, with each VS check.
7. Assess clotting factors, along with other lab results.
8. Notify MD for changes in assessment, VS, hemodynamics, access site, pulses, EKG, pain, or lab results.
9. Do not elevate the head of the bed >30°.
10. Maintain immobilization of the extremity where the access site is located.
11. Administer antiemetics, PRN, as ordered.
12. Provide patient/family education and emotional support.
13. Reposition the patient every 2 hours.
14. Encourage coughing and deep breathing, if applicable.
15. Continue to hold metformin (Glucophage) ×48 hours.

The arterial access site must be closely monitored. A closure device, such as an Angio-Seal™ or a Perclose™, may be used to plug or suture the site. Manual pressure may have been employed to attain hemostasis. Even when the sheath has been removed, the site still holds the potential for oozing, ecchymosis, hematoma development, and/or retroperitoneal bleeding.

If a hematoma develops, apply direct pressure to the site, manually. Perform this for approximately 10 to 15 minutes. Outline the borders of the hematoma with a skin marker and continue frequent site assessments. Back pain can be an indication of retroperitoneal bleeding. Investigate any patient complaints of back and/or groin pain.

If the arterial sheath is left in place post-procedure, it becomes the responsibility of the ICU nurse to discontinue it. The following steps are required for proper arterial sheath removal:

1. Confirm MD order and patient identify via two identifiers.
2. Educate the patient/family.
3. Prep site, per facility policy, for sheath removal.
4. Aspirate 5 to 10 ml of blood from the sheath.
5. Put on sterile gloves.
6. Remove sutures, if applicable.
7. Remove the sheath in one swift movement, while performing step 8.
8. Apply direct pressure, 1 inch above the insertion site until hemostasis. Most nurses find that the index and middle fingers provide the most direct pressure.
9. It may take 15 to 20 minutes, or longer, to achieve hemostasis.
10. Pressure is applied to obtain hemostasis but should not interrupt the distal pulse.
11. Closely monitor the EKG during this time.
12. Monitor VS and peripheral pulses frequently.
13. Apply a sterile dressing to the site.
14. Some facility protocols recommend applying a pressure dressing, fem-stop, or sandbag post-sheath removal.
15. Maintain extremity immobilization per facility protocol, generally 6 hours after sheath removal.
16. Continue frequent monitoring of site and patient.

(Adapted from Chohan & Munden, 2007; Ehlers, 2007; Nettina, 2010; Stillwell, 2006.)

Sheath removal can cause a vagal response, resulting in a slow heart rate and reduced BP. A fluid challenge, or the administration of 0.5 mg atropine, will often improve the situation. Administer both, as ordered. Be prepared for such situations prior to sheath removal. Alert another health care team member when removing a sheath.

===============*FAST FACTS in a NUTSHELL*

Complications related to cardiac catheterization are arrhythmias, bleeding, pericardial effusion, cardiac tamponade, dysrhythmias, embolus, endocarditis, issues regarding peripheral pulses, access site or retroperitoneal hematoma formation, myocardial infarction, pulmonary edema, reactions to the contrast dye, thrombus, stroke, and vaso-vagal response.

ELECTROPHYSIOLOGY STUDY

An electrophysiology study (EPS) is generally performed in the same area as a cardiac catheterization. **During this procedure, the electrical system of the heart is tested. Venous access is required.** The femoral, subclavian, internal jugular, and/or median cephalic veins are used. Sheaths are inserted, and catheters, guided by fluoroscopy, are directed into the right atrium, right ventricle, and, possibly, the left atrium.

The procedure is performed with aseptic technique, and with moderate "conscious" sedation. Rarely, general anesthesia is employed. Anticoagulation may be initiated, depending on the procedure.

If abnormalities are found in the electrical conduction system of the heart, an ablation, pacemaker, or internal cardiac defibrillator may be completed/inserted. Complications related to EPS are similar to those of cardiac catheterization.

Patient preparation for an EPS is similar to that for cardiac catheterization. However, some additional medications, such as beta-blockers, are held prior to the procedure. **Confirm orders with the physician.** Post-procedural monitoring and implementations are basically the same as a cardiac catheterization, with the exception of the sheaths.

If venous sheaths are to be removed in the ICU, follow the same steps as for an arterial sheath removal, but apply

direct pressure 1 inch below the sheath insertion site. If both femoral veins have a sheath, remove one side at a time. If two sheaths are noted in one vein, remove both simultaneously. When removing a venous sheath from the neck, position the head of the bed at least 30°, if possible.

POST-CABG PATIENTS

Preparing a patient for CABG is somewhat similar to that for a cardiac catheterization. Pre-operative skin and oral care are ordered. NPO status is strict, per anesthesia guidelines. **Confirm both per physician's order.**

Patients recovering from a CABG are generally cared for in a cardiovascular intensive care unit (CVICU). They are received from the OR while still under the effects of general anesthesia. The highly specialized nurses in this unit work together as a team to receive the report, assess the patient, apply patient warming methods, and connect the in-room ventilator, monitors, and suction, along with any other required devices.

A post-CABG patient will already be intubated. A nasogastric or orogastric tube, epicardial pacing wires, mediastinal chest tubes, pleural tubes, PA catheter, arterial line, and urinary catheter will be in place. Dressings will cover the sternotomy site and saphenous vein harvesting sites. A radial artery is infrequently harvested.

The patient will be unresponsive, immediately post-op, because of anesthesia. Several IV drips, fluids, and blood products may be infusing to stabilize hemodynamics.

All this activity seems daunting, yet **most patients wean quickly from the ventilator and medications.** As the effect of anesthesia wanes, they become arousable. This recovery period is challenging and rewarding. Occasionally, a patient will require continued vasoactive medications, IABP therapy, sustained ventilation assistance, and in a worst-case scenario, a return trip to the OR to evaluate excessive bleeding or relieve tamponade.

General guidelines for the recovery of post-CABG patients include:

- Performance of a complete physical assessment upon arrival to unit; see Chapter 5 for details.
- Continuous monitoring of VS, hemodynamics, and EKG.
- Hourly assessment of neuro status, chest tube drainage, heart tones, respiratory status, incision sites, peripheral pulses, and urine output.
- Maintain SBP between 100 and 120 mmHG and MAP >70, via vasoactive drips and IV fluid, as ordered.
- Monitor lab work; notify MD of abnormal results.
- Check and treat blood glucose, as ordered.
- Administer blood and blood products, as ordered, per facility protocol.
- Notify MD for CT drainage >100 ml over 2 hours.
- Administer electrolyte therapy, as ordered.
- Warm patient to approximately 37°C.
- Manage pain adequately.
- Administer medications for agitation/restlessness, PRN, as ordered.
- Suction, PRN.
- Assess ETT placement, at least once per shift.
- Wean patient, per protocol, from ventilator; see Chapter 10 for guidelines.
- Once extubated, encourage coughing and deep breathing, along with incentive spirometry use.
- Perform chest tube care; refer to Chapter 14. Mediastinal tubes may be gently milked, if ordered by the MD. Do not milk a pleural tube.
- Assist with chest removal, when needed; refer to Chapter 14 for guidelines.
- For temporary pacing via epicardial wires and wire care, refer to Chapter 13.
- Removal of epicardial wires is completed by an advanced practioner, at the bedside. A sterile occlusive dressing will cover the site.
- Confirm completion of a post-op chest x-ray.

- Anticipate daily chest x-ray.
- Turn the patient every 2 hours.
- Provide frequent patient re-orientation.
- Perform/assist with ROM exercises.
- The morning after surgery, ambulate the patient to a chair, if applicable. Expect a temporary increase in chest tube drainage with the first ambulation.
- Complete sternal, leg/arm incision care once a day, per facility guidelines.
- Apply sequentional compression devices, as ordered.
- Provide frequent patient/ family education and emotional support.
- Consult physical therapy, occupational therapy, and other members of the health care team early to improve patient outcomes.
- Follow ACLS protocol, if required.

(Adapted from Chohan & Munden, 2007; Nettina, 2010; Stillwell, 2006.)

===============================*FAST FACTS in a NUTSHELL*

Medications frequently administered and/or titrated to maintain hemodynamics within physician-specified parameters are dobutamine (Dobutrex), dopamine, epinephrine, milrinone (Primacor), nitroglycerin, nitroprusside (Nipride), vasopressin (Pitressin), isoproterenol (Isuprel), and norepinephrine (Levophed).

Some post-CABG patients require left atrial pressure (LAP) monitoring. This device measures left ventricular function, overall cardiovascular status, and offers another look at hemodynamics.

The catheter is inserted into the left atrium (LA) during surgery. It is brought through the superior pulmonary vein into the LA. An incision is made in the mediastinum, and the other end of the catheter is pulled through the skin. It is connected to a transducer, and the waveform is monitored similarly to a PA catheter. An in-line air filter is used to reduce the risk of air embolus.

A normal LAP reading is 4 to 12 mmHg, read in mean. The catheter should not be flushed. The air port of the transducer must be level with the phlebostatic axis. The pressure is recorded at end-expiration. The transducer should be re-leveled with patient positioning.

Troubleshooting is similar to that for a PA catheter, with the exception of a NO flushing rule for an LAP. If the waveform appears dampened, try to aspirate blood. If it remains damp, notify the physician and anticipate catheter removal. The LAP should not be used to draw blood or administer medications.

Closely monitor the EKG for ventricular dysrhythmias when an LAP is in place. Notify the physician of changes in the reading. Care of the exit site is similar to that for a PA catheter site.

LAP removal is generally performed by an advanced practioner 24 to 48 hours after surgery. Leaving it in longer increases the risk of an air embolus. Mediastinal chest tubes should be maintained at least 2 hours post-LAP removal, as bleeding into the mediastinal area is possible. A sterile, occlusive dressing is applied to the site.

Once the LAP is removed, monitor the site for bleeding. **Frequently assess the patient for the signs and symptoms of a cardiac tamponade.**

═══════════════════════════*FAST FACTS in a NUTSHELL*

Complications of CABG include arrhythmias, pericardial effusion, cardiac tamponade, dysrhythmias, fluid/electrolyte imbalances, gastrointestinal dysfunction, hemorrhage, hypertension or hypotension, myocardial infarction, renal failure, respiratory failure, and stroke.

Cardiac valve replacement/repair, septal defect repair, and other cardiac surgery patients having undergone a sternotomy require comparable post-operative care. The complications from these types of surgeries are similar to those of CABG.

Transplant Patients

INTRODUCTION

There are over 100,000 candidates on the organ transplant waiting list right now. While this number is small compared to the number of patients diagnosed with cardiovascular disease, the care and recovery of transplant recipients remains a vital subject.

Multiple organs and body components can be transplanted. Recipients requiring ICU stays include: cardiac, liver, lung, pancreas, and renal transplant patients.

In this chapter you will learn:

1. General guidelines for the recovery of organ transplant recipients.
2. The signs, symptoms, and potential treatment of transplant rejection.
3. Guidelines specific to cardiac, liver, lung, pancreas, and renal transplant patients.

RECOVERY GUIDELINES FOR ORGAN TRANSPLANT RECIPIENTS

Many types of organ transplants occur in the United States each year. Before being placed on the United Network for

Organ Sharing (UNOS) waiting list, a patient undergoes rigorous testing. Once the criteria for becoming a recipient are met, the patient is placed on the list and...waits. When a suitable match is found, the patient is prepped per protocol and the particular organ transplant surgery is performed.

The following implementations apply to most organ transplant recipients cared for in the ICU:

- Reverse isolation precautions, per facility policy.
- Complete head-to-toe assessment upon arrival to unit.
- Continuous monitoring of respiratory status, SaO_2, SpO_2, and ABGs.
- Frequent physical and neuro re-assessment.
- Continuous monitoring of the EKG for changes; arrhythmias and dysrhythmias are common.
- Frequent monitoring of hemodynamics.
- Titrate vasoactive drips to maintain VS and hemodynamics within ordered parameters.
- Ongoing assessment of fluid status; calculating fluid balance every 12 hours.
- Administer diuretics, as ordered, to prevent fluid overload.
- Maintain aseptic technique during IV and CVL site care and dressing changes.
- Document amount and appearance of chest tube drainage.
- Notify MD of chest tube drainage >200 ml in 1 hour.
- Record input and output each shift.
- Assess lab values. Notify MD of abnormal results.
- Warm patient to approximately 37°C.
- Assess for signs/symptoms of infection.
- Manage pain adequately.
- Infuse leukocyte depleted, cytomegalovirus-negative blood and blood products, as ordered, per facility protocol.
- Ensure completion of a daily chest x-ray.
- Wean from the ventilator, per MD order. The extubation goal, for most transplant patients, is within 24 hours post-op.

- Use chest physiotherapy, incentive spirometry, and postural drainage; encourage coughing and deep breathing after extubation.
- Educate the patient regarding splinting of incision.
- Administer H2 blockers or proton pump inhibitors, as ordered.
- Evaluate gastrointestinal (GI) status for possible paralytic ileus.
- Expect the initiation of enteral feedings, once bowel sounds return.
- Complete a daily weight.
- Administer antibiotics, antifungals, and antivirals, as ordered.
- Administer immunosuppressive medications, as ordered. Examples include
  - Alemtuzumab (Campath)
  - Azathioprine (Imuran)
  - Corticosteroids
  - Cychlophosphamide (Cytoxan)
  - Cyclosporine (Gengraf)
  - Mycophenolate mofetil (MMF)
  - Sirolimus (Rapamune)
  - Tacrolimus (FK-506)
- Review serum immunosuppressive drug levels. Determine whether they are within therapeutic range and notify MD.
- Assess for signs and symptoms of acute rejection, such as fever, headache, nausea, vomiting, chills, malaise, and increased weight.
- With suspicion of rejection, anticipate an organ biopsy.
- Elevate the head of the bed 30°, unless contraindicated.
- Turn the patient every 2 hours, unless contraindicated.
- Provide, or assist with, proper oral care.
- Perform ROM exercises, as tolerated.
- Encourage mobilization and ambulation early, as tolerated.
- Consult a nutritionist, physical therapist, occupational therapist, wound care specialist, and other members of the health care team early.

- Every transplant recipient requires much post-op education, emotional support, and medical follow-up.

==*FAST FACTS in a NUTSHELL*

Immunosuppressive therapy has the potential to produce toxic side effects in almost every system of the body. Examples of how such toxicity might present include: elevated blood glucose, coma, confusion, cortical blindness, encephalopathy, gingival hyperplasia, hyperkalemia, hypertension, leukopenia, quadriplegia, seizures, and tremors. Complications related to organ transplants include: atelectasis, hemorrhage, infection, organ(s) rejection, paralytic ileus, pneumonia, renal failure, bleeding, and thrombosis.

(Adapted from Alspach, 2006; Collins & Johnston, 2009; Nettina, 2010; Rudow & Goldstein, 2008; Stillwell, 2006; Wyckoff et al., 2009.)

REJECTION

Organ rejection can occur following any type of transplant. There are four major categories of organ rejection: hyperacute, accelerated, acute T-cell mediated, and chronic. Each category is treated differently, according to the underlying cause and symptoms.

The general symptoms associated with rejection are chills, diaphoresis, fever, exhaustion, hypertension, increased weight gain, poor appetite, tenderness at graft site, peripheral edema, and a drop in urine output. Lab results and diagnostic test results vary with the organ transplanted.

Hyperacute rejection happens almost immediately following the transplant and is often untreatable. Accelerated rejection happens within 2 to 5 days following the transplant and is managed with plasmapheresis and immunoglobulin G administration. Steroid and/or increased immunosuppression therapy is used to treat acute T-cell medicated rejection, which takes place within a few days to a few weeks following the transplant. Rejection that occurs months to a year from the time of the transplant is generally chronic and not reversible. A gradual loss in organ/graft function is seen.

ORGAN-SPECIFIC TRANSPLANT RECOVERY GUIDELINES

Lung

- Frequent lung auscultation.
- Assess airway pressures and tidal volume, while intubated.
- Only suction with a pre-measured suction catheter whose length has been approved, according to OR measurements during surgery. This allows avoidance of surgical suture lines.
- A bronchoscopy may be required to observe and remove secretions.
- Anticipate the administration of Prostaglandin E1 via IV or nitric oxide via inhalation, as ordered, for recipients with a history of pulmonary hypertension.
- Place a single-lung recipient in the lateral decubitus position with the native lung down and the new lung up. The exception to this rule is during acute rejection. Then, the native lung should be up.
- Place a double-lung recipient supine for 6 to 8 hours, or until stable, then initiate position changes.
- The MD may order a continuous lateral rotation bed.

(Adapted from Alspach, 2006; Nettina, 2010; Stillwell, 2006; Wyckoff et al., 2009.)

═══════════════════════════*FAST FACTS in a NUTSHELL*

Complications related specifically to lung transplants include abnormal gas exchange, alveolar and interstitial infiltrates, decreased lung compliance, and pulmonary edema.

Heart

- Following heart transplantation, the heart is denervated. It will not respond to autonomic nervous system stimulation. The heart rate will not change in response to stress, decreased cardiac output, or atropine.
- Assess for signs/symptoms of cardiac tamponade.
- Closely monitor the EKG. A high potential for the development of a junctional rhythm, or AV block, exists.
- Perform cardiac pacing, as needed.
- Administer prostaglandins, as ordered, to lower pulmonary vascular resistance.
- Expect a minimal amount of right ventricular dysfunction.

(Adapted from Alspach, 2006; Nettina, 2010; Stillwell, 2006; Wyckoff et al., 2009.)

═══════════════════════════*FAST FACTS in a NUTSHELL*

Hyperacute rejection is not common following cardiac transplant. Signs and symptoms of rejection, or graft failure, are arrhythmias, coronary artery occlusions, hypotension, cardiogenic shock, and ventricular failure.Complications specific to heart transplants include pericardial effusion, cardiac tamponade, embolism, HTN, myocardial infarction, respiratory failure, stroke, and tricuspid regurgitation.

Liver

- Closely monitor BP, as hypertension is common.
- Administer medications, such as labetalol (Trandate) PRN, as ordered.
- Frequently assess the GI system. Note ascites, bowel sounds, tenderness, nausea, vomiting, and distension.
- Assess nasogastric (NG) tube frequently and maintain patency.

- Do not re-position, or irrigate, the NG tube without an MD order.
- Monitor amount and appearance of bile. Normal bile is thick, viscous, and dark gold to brown in color. Notify MD of changes.
- Obtain abdominal girth every 12 hours.
- Monitor liver function tests (LFTs), fibrinogen level, clotting factors, BG, and K+ levels closely.
- Administer insulin, as ordered.
- Frequently assess acid-base balance.
- Anticipate a Doppler ultrasound, within 24 hours post-op, to assess transplant site.
- Assess for fever, jaundice, shoulder pain, sepsis, and changes in drainage from incisions and drains, as these symptoms can be indicative of a biliary leak.
- Assess for jaundice, itching, abnormal bilirubin and/or alkaline phosphatase, as these symptoms can be indicative of a biliary stricture.
- Perform oral care with nystatin, as ordered.
- When the patient is able to tolerate PO intake, encourage a high-protein diet.

(Adapted from Alspach, 2006; Nettina, 2010; Rudow & Goldstein, 2008; Stillwell, 2006; Wyckoff et al., 2009.)

====*FAST FACTS in a NUTSHELL*

- Signs and symptoms specific to a liver transplant rejection are elevated LFTs and hyperbilirubinemia.
- Primary non-function is the term used for liver graft failure occurring immediately post-op. The patient can become comatose and exhibit extreme coagulopathy, severely reduced urine output, jaundice, and/or very low BG. Another transplant is the only way to reverse the condition.
- Complications specific to liver transplants include: aphasia, acute liver failure, encephalopathy, myelinlysis biliary complications, and neuropathy.

Pancreas

- Frequent assessment of GI system.
- Assess NG tube frequently and maintain patency.
- Do not re-position or irrigate the NG tube without an MD order.
- Palpate graft site for swelling, tenderness, and pain.
- Check BG every hour.
- Titrate insulin drip per MD parameters.
- Titrate 50% dextrose infusion, if applicable, per MD order.
- Check urine amylase, lipase, and pH every 6 hours.
- Monitor acid-base balance.
- Administer bicarbonate, as ordered.
- Give anticoagulants, as ordered.
- Assess for lower abdominal pain, fever, leukocytosis, and elevated serum amylase and/or creatinine, as these symptoms can be indicative of an anastomotic leak.
- Complete bed rest, without hip flexion on the side of the graft, for 48 to 72 hours post-op.

(Adapted from Alspach, 2006; Collins and Johnston, 2009; Nettina, 2010; Stillwell, 2006; Wyckoff et al., 2009.)

==*FAST FACTS in a NUTSHELL*

Signs and symptoms specific to a pancreatic transplant rejection include: elevated amylase and lipase. Complications specific to pancreas transplants include: acute pancreatitis, anastomotic leaks, and urethritis in male patients.

Over 90% of pancreas transplants occur with kidney transplants because the recipient also suffers from end-stage renal disease.

Kidney

- Uncomplicated cases may go from the recovery room directly to the floor.

- Fluid management, with ½ normal saline, is often performed based on a 1 ml of urine output for 1 ml of fluid replacement scale (Wyckoff et al., 2009; Houghton & LePage, 2009).
- Administer furosemide (Lasix) drips, as ordered, generally 5 to 20 mg/hour.
- Administer low-dose dopamine, as ordered, usually 2 to 5 mcg/kg/min.
- Treat hypertension, per MD orders.
- Check BG every hour.
- Titrate insulin infusion via MD parameters.
- Closely monitor K+ levels.
- Administer bicarbonate, as ordered, to manage renal tubular acidosis.
- Assess for pain over transplant site and thick, yellow drainage from the incision site; both can be indicative of a urine leak.
- Anticipate a renal ultrasound on post-op day 1.
- Complete bed rest, without hip flexion on the side of the graft, for 48 to 72 hours post-op.

(Adapted from Alspach, 2006; Collins and Johnston, 2009; Nettina, 2010; Stillwell, 2006; Wyckoff et al., 2009.)

═══════════════════════*FAST FACTS in a NUTSHELL*

Signs and symptoms specific to renal transplant rejection include elevated creatinine and increased BUN. Complications specific to kidney transplants include lymphocele development, thrombosis, ureteral obstruction, and the development of a urine leak.

18

Burn Unit Basics

INTRODUCTION

According to the American Burn Association, approximately 45,000 patients were hospitalized in 2010 for the treatment of burns. A little over half were treated at specialized burn centers, and the remaining 20,000 patients were treated at regular facilities. These statistics and the fact that the integumentary system is the largest organ of the human body make education and skills regarding burn care an essential part of every ICU.

In this chapter you will learn:

1. The types of burns.
2. A description of the rule of nines.
3. The classification guidelines for burns and corresponding nursing implementations.
4. The signs and symptoms of smoke inhalation and carbon monoxide poisoning.

BASIC BURN BREAKDOWN

A burn is simply a breakdown of the skin. **The major types of burns are chemical, electrical, radiation, scald, and thermal**

burns. The severity of a burn is based on the percentage of body surface area (BSA) affected, the depth of the wound, the patient's age, the area of the body burned, the patient's medical history, accompanying injuries/issues, and the existence of an inhalation injury. Severity also increases with wounds to the eyes, ears, face, hands, feet, and groin.

THE RULE OF NINES

The determination of BSA involved in a burn is often done **by the rule of nines, in which the body is broken down into percentage areas that are assessed for wounds.** Once the assessment is complete, the total BSA affected can be calculated.

═══════════════════════════════════════*FAST FACTS in a NUTSHELL*

Accepted percentages according to the rule of nines:

- Face, back of head: 4.5% each
- Groin: 1%
- Low back (buttocks): 9%
- Palms: 1% each
- Chest, back: 9% each
- Front or back of each arm: 4.5% each
- Abdomen: 9%
- Front or back of each leg: 9% each

(Adapted from Burn percentage in Adults, 2008; Nettina, 2010; Stillwell, 2006.)

An example of a burn BSA calculation by the rule of nines is a case in which the front of one leg (9%), the groin (1%), and the abdomen (9%) are burned. The total BSA involved is 19%.

BURN CLASSIFICATION

Burns were once classified as being 1st, 2nd, or 3rd degree. This has been changed to four categories that are characterized by wound depth.

- *Superficial:* Painful. Pink/red skin, no blistering, possible minimal edema, blanching. Epidermis is affected. Heals in 3–5 days; no scar.
- *Partial thickness:* Painful. Pink/red skin, blisters, weepy skin, blanching. Epidermis and superficial dermis affected. Heals in 2–3 weeks; possible scarring.
- *Deep partial thickness:* Painful. Pink/white dry skin, possible blisters, no blanching. Epidermis, superficial dermis, and deep dermis affected. Heals in 3–6 weeks; possible scarring.
- *Full thickness:* Actual wound is pain-free but surrounding area aches. Red/white/brown/black dry, leathery skin, no blistering. All layers of the skin and subcutaneous tissue are affected; may include muscle, tendon, and/or bone. Eschar will need to be removed. Heals in >1 month and typically requires grafting. Scarring will occur.

(Adapted from Alspach, 2006; Buettner, 2010; Chohan & Munden, 2007; Nettina, 2010; Stillwell, 2006; Wyckoff et al., 2009.)

TYPES OF BURNS

Chemical burns can cause tissue oxidation and denaturation, cellular dehydration and coagulation, and/or blistering. The symptoms are burning, pain, swelling, fluid loss, and/or discoloration. The severity and type of injury varies with the type of chemical exposure.

Electrical burns present with various symptoms. There may be white and/or leathery charring at the entrance and exit sites of the wound, the smell of burned skin, minimal or no pain, visual changes, seizures, and/or paralysis. EKG changes, such as ventricular fibrillation, asystole, nonspecific ST-segment changes, and sinus tachycardia, are often observed. Spinal cord trauma is possible. Rhabdomyolosis may be present. The iceberg effect—small wound sites with a large amount of internal damage—is often noted.

Radiation burns are not common. These injuries affect DNA and have a long-term effect. The immediate injury site exhibits characteristics similar to a wound.

Scalds occur from contact with hot steam or liquid. Children are most commonly treated for this type of burn. The appearance of such wounds ties in closely with the classification descriptions.

Flames, or contact with something extremely hot, cause thermal burns. These wounds fit the classification descriptions very closely.

INHALATION ISSUES

An inhalation injury from steam, smoke, or chemicals is frequently characterized by shortness of breath, hoarseness, chest tightness, rapid respirations, singed nares, gray or black sputum, facial burns, and/or stridor.

Carbon monoxide poisoning is characterized by hallmark cherry-red skin. Symptoms also include confusion, nausea, syncope, headache, changes in vision, and an increased carboxyhemoglobin (COHb) level (generally >10%). Carbon monoxide poisoning is often experienced when smoke exposure occurred in a small, confined area. Severe cases may be treated with hyperbaric oxygen.

═══════════════════════════════════*FAST FACTS in a NUTSHELL*

Burn victims cared for in the ICU usually meet the following criteria:

- Over 20% total BSA effected
- Full thickness burns
- Co-morbidities, such as cardiovascular disease, diabetes, or kidney disease
- Inhalation or high-voltage electrical injury
- Additional injuries requiring ICU intervention

GENERAL BURN CARE GUIDELINES

Complications associated with burns can be severe, including shock, kidney failure, respiratory distress/failure, sepsis, and limb loss. **Burn management is focused on complication prevention.** The following are guidelines and implementations for ICU burn treatment:

- Continuous monitoring of VS, EKG, and hemodynamics
- Maintain mean arterial pressure >60 via fluid infusion or vasoactive medication administration, as ordered
- Continuous monitoring of SpO_2
- Maintain SpO_2 >95%
- Assess ABG results
- For patients with elevated COHb levels, provide 100% O_2 therapy, as ordered
- Anticipate intubation, PRN. Mechanical ventilation is often low volume, 5–8 ml/kg
- Suction, PRN
- Assess sputum for color, thickness, and odor
- Administer bronchodilators, as ordered
- Perform chest physiotherapy, as ordered
- Ensure chest x-ray completion
- Encourage cough and deep breathing; and incentive spirometry, if applicable
- Be alert to the possible development of laryngeal edema up to 72 hours post-injury
- Perform a complete head-to-toe assessment upon arrival to unit. Refer to Chapter 5 for guidelines
- Perform frequent re-assessments. Notify the physician of changes
- Maintain a patent IV
- Anticipate the insertion of a CVL and/or PA catheter
- Lactated Ringer's at 2–4 ml × weight in kg × % of BSA burned is generally instituted, starting from the time of injury:
  ○ 1st half infused within 8 hours
  ○ 2nd half infused over the following 16 hours
- No colloids given during the first 24 hours post-injury
- During the second 24 hours post-injury, colloids are usually infused at 0.5 ml of colloid × weight in kg × % of BSA burned

- 2000 ml D5W, infused over 24 hours, is often added to the second 24-hour post-injury period
- Administer blood/blood products, as ordered, per facility protocol
- Closely monitor fluid status; measure input and output every hour
- Placement of a nasogastric tube, as ordered
- Test gastric pH. Assess for blood in emesis, nasogastric drainage, and/or stool
- Administer H_2 antagonists, proton pump inhibitors, and antacids, as ordered
- Insert urinary catheter, using aseptic technique
- Assess urine appearance. Notify the physician of changes in color
- Urine output should be 30–50 ml/hour for most burn victims
- Urine output for electrical burn victims should be >100 cc/hour
- Observe for the signs/symptoms of abdominal compartment syndrome, such as poor ventilation and reduced urine output during fluid administration
- Complete a daily weight
- Assess lab work such as albumin, blood glucose, BUN, creatinine, hematocrit, hemoglobin, K+, osmolality, partial prothrombin time, protime, urine specific gravity, and WBC
- Frequently assess peripheral pulses and neurovascular status
- Doppler extremity pulses, PRN
- Manage pain effectively
- Anticipate the use of a PCA pump for alert/oriented patients
- Administer anxiolytic medications, as ordered
- For a chemical burn, ensure complete removal of the chemical from body. Do not rub skin; blot or brush
- Pre-medicate patient prior to wound care
- Perform wound care daily, or twice a day, as ordered:
  - Cleanse and debride, as ordered, using aseptic technique

- ○ Clip hair around site
- ○ Dress, as ordered. Wounds may be left open, or closed (covered with a topical medication and dressed)
- Topical medications that may be ordered are:
  - ○ Silver sulfadiazine 1% (Silvadene)
  - ○ Mafenide Acetate 5% or 10% (Sulfamylon)
  - ○ Silver nitrate 0.5%
  - ○ Silver sheeting (Acticoat)
  - ○ Mupirocin (Bactroban)
- Assess burn site for drainage. Document appearance, color, and odor
- Assess wound for changes in appearance, margins, or drainage
- Perform wound culture, as ordered
- Cover partial thickness wounds to reduce pain
- An escharotomy, or fasciotomy, may be indicated for full thickness and/or circumferential burns
- Wound excision and/or skin grafting may be performed
- Artificial skin products may be used
- Review medical history for tetanus administration. If none is found, administer tetanus shot, as ordered
- Re-position/assist with position changes at least every 2 hours
- Maintain room temperature between 85 and 90°F
- Maintain the head of the bed at least 30 degrees, if not contraindicated
- Perform/assist with ROM exercises to prevent contractures
- Maintain contact isolation precautions, as indicated per facility protocol
- Perform frequent hand hygiene
- Do not share equipment such as stethoscopes, thermometers, or BP cuffs among patients
- Provide enhanced nutrition related to increased energy needs for healing
- Consult nutritionist, physical therapist, occupational therapist, psychiatrist, social services, and other members of the health care team early to improve patient outcomes

- Provide frequent patient/family education and emotional support

(Adapted from Alspach, 2006; Buettner, 2010; Chohan & Munden, 2007; Ehlers, 2007; Nettina, 2010; Stillwell, 2006; Wyckoff et al., 2009.)

Appendix A: "Do Not Use" List for Abbreviations, Acronyms, and Symbols

Do Not Use	Potential Problem	Use Instead
U (unit)	Mistaken for "0" (zero), the number "4" (four), or "cc"	Write "unit"
IU (international unit)	Mistaken for IV (intravenous) or the number 10 (ten)	Write "international unit"
Q.D., QD, q.d., qd (daily)	Mistaken for each other.	Write "daily"
Q.O.D., QOD, q.o.d, qod (every other day)	Period after the Q mistaken for "I" and the "0" mistaken for "I"	Write "every other day"
Trailing zero (X.0 mg)*	Decimal point is missed	Write X mg
Lack of leading zero (.X mg)		Write 0.X mg
MS	Can mean morphine sulfate or magnesium sulfate	Write "morphine sulfate" / Write "magnesium sulfate"

MSO$_4$ and MSO$_4$	Confused with one another	
> (Greater than)	Misinterpreted as the number "7" (seven) or the letter "L."	Write "greater than"
< (Less than)		Write "less than"
	Confused with one another	
Abbreviations for drug names	Misinterpreted due to similar abbreviations for multiple drugs	Write drug names in full
Apothecary units	Unfamiliar to many Practitioners. Confused with metric units	Use metric units
@	Mistaken for the number "2" (two)	Write "at"
cc	Mistaken for U (units) when poorly written	Write "mL" or "ml" or "milliliters"
µg	Mistaken for mg (milligrams)	Write "mcg" or "micrograms"

* Exception: A "trailing zero" may be used only where required to demonstrate the level of precision of the value being reported, such as for laboratory results, imaging studies that report the size of lesions, or catheter tube sizes. It may not be used in medication orders or other medication-related documentation.

RESOURCES

Facts about the Official "Do Not Use" List. Retrieved May 1, 2011, from www.jointcommission.org/assets/1/18/Official_Do%20 Not%20Use_List_%206_10.pdf

ISMP's List of Error-Prone Abbreviations, Symbols, and Dose Designations. Retrieved May 9, 2011, from www.ismp.org/tools/ errorproneabbreviations.pdf

Springhill Medical Center. (2009). *Unsafe Abbreviationtions.* Mobile, AL: Author.

Appendix B: Basic EKG Rhythm Examples

SINUS RHYTHM

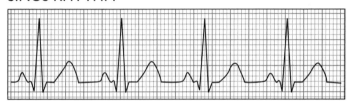

SINUS BRADYCARDIA

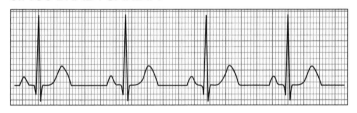

SINUS TACHYCARDIA

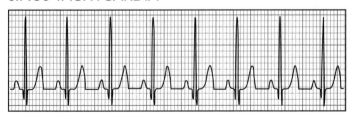

FIRST DEGREE HEART BLOCK

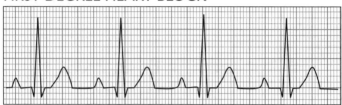

SECOND DEGREE HEART BLOCK, TYPE I
WENCKEBACH

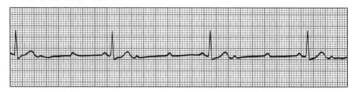

SECOND DEGREE HEART BLOCK, TYPE II

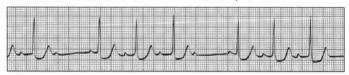

THIRD DEGREE HEART BLOCK

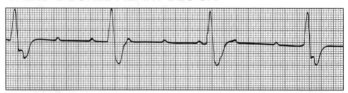

ATRIAL FLUTTER

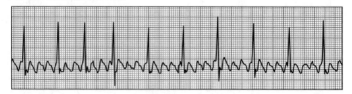

ATRIAL FIBRILLATION

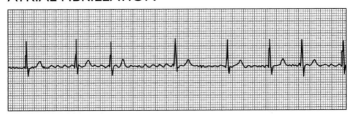

JUNCTIONAL

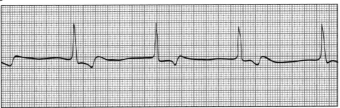

SUPRAVENTRICULAR TACHYCARDIA

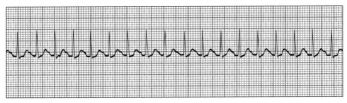

PAROXYSMAL SUPRAVENTRICULAR TACHYCARDIA

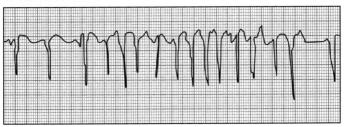

IDIOVENTRICULAR

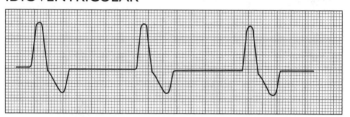

SINUS RHYTHM WITH UNIFOCAL PVCS

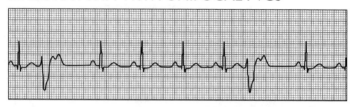

SINUS RHYTHM WITH MULTIFOCAL PVCS

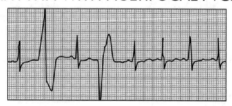

BIGEMINAL PVCS

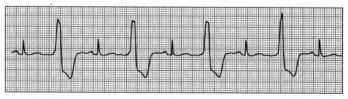

VENTRICULAR TACHYCARDIA

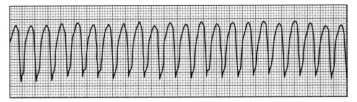

VENTRICULAR FIBRILLATION

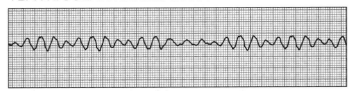

VENTRICULAR PACING

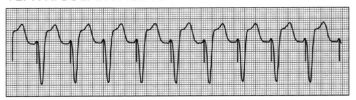

ASYSTOLE

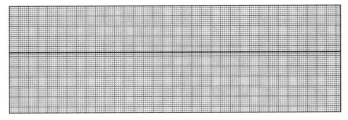

Appendix C: 12 Lead EKG Electrode Placement

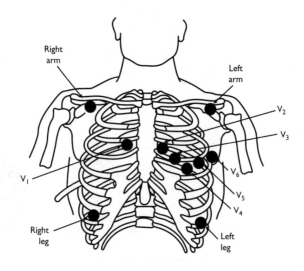

ELECTRODE PLACEMENT

1. Left arm: Left deltoid or wrist
2. Right arm: Right deltoid or wrist
3. Left leg: Left thigh or ankle
4. Right leg: Right thigh or ankle
5. V1: 4th intercostal space at the right sternal border
6. V2: 4th intercostal space at the left sternal border
7. V3: Midway between V2 and V4
8. V4: Midclavicular line at the 5th intercostal space
9. V5: Anterior axillary line at the 5th intercostal space
10. V6: Midaxillary line at the 5th intercostal space

Appendix D: Normal Hemodynamic Values and Vital Signs

Abbreviation	Parameter	Normal Range
PAS	Pulmonary artery systolic	15–30 mmHg
PAD	Pulmonary artery diastolic	5–15 mmHg
PAWP (PCWP)	Pulmonary artery wedge pressure (Pulmonary capillary wedge pressure)	4–12 mmHg
CVP (RAP)	Central venous pressure (Right atrial pressure)	2–6 mmHg
MAP	Mean arterial pressure	70–105 mmHg
CO	Cardiac output	4–8 L/min
CI	Cardiac index	2.5–4.0 L/min/m^2
SV	Stroke volume	60–120 mL/beat
SI	Stroke index	30–65 mL/beat/m^2
LVSWI	Left ventricular stroke work index	40–70 g–m/m^2
RVSWI	Right ventricular stroke work index	5–12 g–m/m^2

PVR	Pulmonary vascular resistance	50–250 dynes/s/cm^{-5}
PVRI	Pulmonary vascular resistance index	45–200 dynes/s/cm^{-5}/m^2
SVR	Systemic vascular resistance	800–1400 dynes/s/cm^{-5}
SVRI	Systemic vascular resistance index	1700–2600 dynes/s/cm^{-5}/m^2
SBP	Systolic blood pressure	90–140 mmHg
DBP	Diastolic blood pressure	50–90 mmHg
HR	Heart rate	60–100 beats/min
Temp	Temperature	97.8–99.1°F 36.5–37.3°C
RR	Respiratory rate	12–20 breaths/min
SvO_2	Mixed venous oxygen saturation	60–80%
SaO_2	Arterial oxygen saturation	≥95%
$ScvO_2$	Central venous oxygen saturation	≥70%

SOURCES

Alspach, J. G. (2006). *Core curriculum for critical care nursing* (6th ed.). St. Louis, MO: Saunders Elsevier.

Fauci, A., Braunwald, E., Kasper, D., Hauser, S., Longo, D., Jameson, J., et al. (2008). *Harrison's principles of internal medicine* (17th ed.). New York: McGraw Hill.

Stillwell, S. B. (2006). *Mosby's critical care nursing reference* (4th ed.). St. Louis, MO: Mosby Elsevier.

Appendix E: List of Abbreviations

ABG	arterial blood gas
A-line	arterial line
AV	arteriovenous
BE	base excess
BG	blood glucose
BIVAD	biventricular assist device
BNP	brain natriuretic peptide
BP	blood pressure
BSA	body surface area
BUN	blood urea nitrogen
CABG	coronary artery bypass graft
CAVH	continuous arteriovenous hemofiltration
CAVHD	continuous arteriovenous hemodialysis
CCL	cardiac catheterization lab
CCU	cardiac care unit
CI	cardiac index
CK	creatinine kinase
CMC	cardiac medicine certification
CO	cardiac output
COHb	carboxyhemoglobin
CPAP	continuous positive airway pressure
CPR	cardiopulmonary resuscitation
CRRT	continuous renal replacement therapy

CSC	cardiac surgery certification
CSF	cerebrospinal fluid
CT	chest tube
CVAD	central venous access device
CVD	cardiovascular disease
CVICU	cardiovascular intensive care unit
CVL	central venous line
CVP	central venous pressure
CVVH	continuous venovenous hemofiltration
CVVHD	continuous venovenous hemodialysis
CVVHDF	continuous venovenous hemodiafiltration
D5	dextrose
DNR	do not resuscitate
DVT	deep vein thrombus
EMAR	electronic medication administration record
EMR	electronic medical record
EN	enteral nutritional
EPS	electrophysiology study
ETT	endotracheal tube
EVD	external ventricular drain
FC	Foley catheter
FIO	fraction of inspired oxygen
FiO_2	oxygen concentration
GCS	Glasgow coma scale
HAI	hospital-acquired infection
HCO_3	bicarbonate
HD	hemodialysis
HEENT	head, eyes, ears, nose, and throat
HEPA	high-efficiency particulate air
HOB	head of bed
IABP	intra-aortic balloon
ICP	intracranial pressure
IMV	intermittent mandatory ventilation
LA	left atrium
LAP	left atrial pressure
LFT	liver function test
LR	lactated Ringer's
LVAD	left ventricular assist device

LVEDP	left ventricular end-diastolic pressure
LVSWI	left ventricular stroke work index
mA	milliamperes
MRA	magnetic resonance angiography
MRI	magnetic resonance imaging
MV	minute volume
MVO_2	myocardial oxygen consumption
NDA	nearing death awareness
NG	naso-gastric
NIBP	noninvasive blood pressure
NICU	neurologic intensive care unit
NPA	Nurse Practice Act
NPO	nothing by mouth
NS	normal saline
NSAID	nonsteroidal anti-inflammatory drug
OPO	organ procurement organization
PA	pulmonary artery
PAD	pulmonary artery diastolic
PAWP	pulmonary artery wedge pressure
PCA	patient controlled analgesia
PCO_2	partial pressure of carbon dioxide
PD	peritoneal dialysis
PEEP	positive-end-expiratory pressure
PEG	percutaneous gastrostomy tube
PET	positron emission tomography
PICC	peripherally inserted central catheter
PIV	peripheral IV
PN	parenteral nutrition
PO	given by mouth
PO_2	partial pressure of oxygen
PPE	personal protective equipment
PPN	peripheral parenteral nutrition
PS	pressure support
RA	right atrium
ROM	range of motion
RR	respiratory rate
RV	right ventricle
SAB	subarachnoid bolt

SaO_2	arterial oxygen saturation
SARS	severe acute respiratory syndrome
SCUF	slow continuous ultrafiltration
SICU	surgical intensive care unit
SIMV	synchronized intermittent mandatory ventilation
SIRS	systemic inflammatory response syndrome
$SjvO_2$	jugular venous oxygen saturation
SPECT	single photon emission tomography
SpO_2	oxyhemoglobin
SpO_2	pulse oximetry
SVC	superior vena cava
SvO_2	mixed-venous oxygen saturation
SVR	systemic venous resistance
TCD	transcranial Doppler
TPN	total parenteral nutrition
UTI	urinary tract infection
VAD	vascular access device
VAD	ventricular assist devices
VAP	ventilator-associated pneumonia
VS	vital signs
VT	tidal volume

References

2.0 early vs. delayed nutrient intake. (2009). Retrieved October 18, 2010, from www.criticalcarenutrition.com/docs/cpg/2.0early_FINAL.pdf

ABIOMED, Inc. (2007, July). Impella 2.5 system, instructions for use. (Document No. 0046–9000 Rev. C.) Retrieved December 2, 2010, from http://www.abiomed.com/products/documents/ImpellaIFU2–080046-9000_rC.pdf

ABIOMED, Inc. (2009). Impella 2.5. Retrieved November 30, 2010, from http:/www.abiomed.com/products/impella.cfm

Alabama Eye Bank. Retrieved on August 3, 2010, from www.alabamaeyebank.org/faq.php

Alexander, M. (Ed.). (2006). Infusion nursing standards of practice. *Journal of Infusion Nursing, 29*(1 Suppl.), S37–S78.

Alspach, J. G. (2006). *Core curriculum for critical care nursing* (6th ed.). St. Louis, MO: Saunders Elsevier.

American Association of Critical-Care Nurses. *About critical care nursing.* Retrieved on April 30, 2010, from classic.aacn.org/AACN/mrkt.nsf/vwdoc/AboutCriticalCareNursing

American Association of Critical-Care Nurses. *Frequently asked questions about CCRN certification.* Retrieved on April 30, 2010, from www.aacn.org/wd/certifications/content/faqsccrn.pcms?menu=certification

American Burn Association. *Burn incidence and treatment in the United States: 2011 fact sheet.* Retrieved on January 9, 2011, from www.ameriburn.org/resources_factsheet.php

American Heart Association. (n.d.). *Cardiovascular disease statistics*. Retrieved on January 5, 2011, from http://www.american-heart.org/presenter.jhtml?identifier=4478

American Medical Directors Association. (2004). *Pain Assessment in Advanced Dementia (PAINAD) Scale*. Retrieved August 14, 2010, from http://www.amda.com/caring/may2004/painad.htm

American Nurses Association. (2002). *Needlestick prevention guide*. Retrieved on November 6, 2010, from www.nuringworld.org/MainMeunCategories/OccupationalandEnvironmental/occupationalhealth/SafeNeedles/NeedlestickPrevention.aspx

American Nurses Association. (2004). *Nursing: Scope and standards of practice*. Washington, DC: Author.

American Nurses Association. *The nursing process: A common thread amongst all nurses*. Retrieved on April 7, 2010, from www.nursingworld.org/EspeciallyForYou/StudentNurses/Thenursingprocess.aspx

Aranky, S., & Aroesty, J. (2010). Medical therapy to prevent perioperative complications after coronary artery bypass graft surgery. In: D. S. Basow (Ed.), *UpToDate*. Waltham, MA: UpToDate.

Ayello, E. A., & Sibbald, R. G. (2008). Preventing pressure ulcers and skin tears. In *Evidence-based geriatric nursing protocols for best practice*. Retrieved on October 18, 2010, from www.guideline.gov/popups/printView.aspx?id=12262

Basic Nursing Assessment. Retrieved on August 22, 2010, from www.medtrng.com/blackboard/basic_nursing_assessment.htm

Beck, B. (2010). *Isolation precaution suggestions*. Mobile, AL: Springhill Medical Center.

Beck, B. (2010). *PPE on-off*. Mobile, AL: Springhill Medical Center.

Bell, L. (Ed.). (2008). *AACN scope and standards for acute and critical care nursing practice* (pp. 10–18). Aliso Viejo, CA: American Association of Critical-Care Nurses.

Brigham and Women's Hospital, Cardiovascular Medicine. (2010, October). Ventricular assist device (VAD). Retrieved on December 21, 2010, from http://www.brighamandwomens.org/Departments_and_Services/medicine/services/cvcenter/Services/ventricular_assist_device/

Buettner, J. R. (2010). *Fast facts for the ER nurse: Emergency room orientation in a nutshell*. New York: Springer Publishing Company.

Burn percentage in adults: Rule of nines. (2008). Retrieved on January 9, 2011, from www.emedicinehealth.com/burn_percentage_in_adults_rule_of_nines/article_em.htm

Calloway, S. D. (2010). *Infection control standards 2010 for the joint commission. Georgia Hospital Association.* Retrieved on October 31, 2010, from www.gha.org/telnet/2595.pdf

Catheterization, female. Retrieved on October 18, 2010, from www.enotes.com/nursing-encyclopedia/catherization-female

Catheterizing the female & male urinary bladder (straight & indwelling). (2007). Retrieved on October 18, 2010, from www.nursingcrib.com/demo-checklist/catheterizing-the-female-male-urinary-bladder-straight-indwelling

Centers for Disease Control and Prevention. (2003). *Guidelines for preventing health-care-associated pneumonia.* Retrieved on October 13, 2010, from www.cdc.gov/mmwr/preview/mmwrhtml/rr5303a1.htm

Centers for Disease Control and Prevention. (2004). *Eye protection for infection control.* Retrieved on November 11, 2010, from www.cdc.gov/niosh/topics/eye/eye-Infectious.html

Centers for Disease Control and Prevention. (2009). *Public health grand rounds.* Retrieved on October 16, 2010, from www.cdc.gov/about/grand-rounds/archives/2009/download/GR-101509.pdf

Centers for Disease Control and Prevention. *Glasgow Coma Scale.* Retrieved on December 26, 2010, from www.cdc.gov/ncipc/pub-res/tbi_toolkit/physicians/gcs.pdf

Chenoweth, C. E. Urinary catheter-related infection and infection prevention systems. *University of Michigan Health System.* Retrieved on September 13, 2010, from www.docstoc.com/docs/476245/Urinary-Catheter-Related-Infections-and-Infection-Prevention-Systems

Chohan, N., & Munden, J. (Eds.). (2007). *Critical care nursing.* Ambler, PA: Lippincott Williams & Wilkins.

Collins, B. H., & Johnston, T. D. (2009). *Renal transplantation (Urology).* Retrieved on January 8, 2011, from http://emedicine.medscape.com/article/430128-print

Cover, M. *New regulations outline content, transmission standards for every American's electronic health records.* Retrieved on July 24, 2010, from cnsnews.com/news/print/69519

Cypel, M., Waddell, T., & Keshavjee, S. (2010). Lung transplantation: Procedure and postoperative management. In: P. Trulock (Ed), *UpToDate*. Waltham, MA: UpToDate.

D'Arcy, Y. (2008). Keep your patient safe during PCA. *Nursing 2008, 38*(1), 50–55. Retrieved November 17, 2010, from www.nursingcenter.com/prodev/cearticleprint.asp?CE_ID= 762689

Datascope Corp. (n.d.). Managing intra-aortic balloon pump therapy. Retrieved December 1, 2010, from http://www.datascope. com/ca/pdf/managing_iabp_therapy.pdf

Ehlers, J. (Ed.). (2007). *AACN's quick reference guide to critical care nursing procedures*. St. Louis, MO: Saunders Elsevier.

Encyclopedia of Surgery. Retrieved on July 26, 2010, from www. surgeryencyclopedia.com/La-Pa/Living-Will.html

Fauci, A., Braunwald, E., Kasper, D., Hauser, S., Longo, D., Jameson, J., et al. (2008). *Harrison's principles of internal medicine* (17th ed.). New York: McGraw Hill Companies, Inc.

Female catheters cause trauma in males. (2010). Retrieved on October 1, 2010, from www.nursingtimes.net/nursing-practice-clinical-research/clinical-subjects/national-patient-safety-agency-rapid-response-reports/female-catheters-cause-trauma-in-males/5015342.article

Foreman, M. D., Milisen, K., & Fulmer, T. T. (Eds.). (2010). *Critical care nursing of older adults: Best practices*. New York: Springer Publishing.

Gaglio, P., & Brown, R. (2010). Overview of medical care of the liver transplant recipient. In: M. Kaplan (Ed), *UpToDate*. Waltham, MA: UpToDate.

Hadaway, L. (2007). Infiltration and extravasation. *American Journal of Nursing, 8*, 61–72.

Hauswirth, K., & Sherk, S. D. (n.d.). Aseptic technique. Retrieved November 1, 2010, www.surgeryencyclopedia.com/A-Ce/Aseptic-Technique.html

Head to toe assessment checklist (older adults). Retrieved on August 15, 2010, from www.allnurses.com/head%20to%20 assessment%20checklist%20older%20adults-1[1]

Heiserman, D. (2008). *Purposes of urinary catheterization*. Retrieved on October 18, 2010, from www.freeed.net/sweethaven/ MedTech/NurseFund/default.asp?INum=3&fraNum=030101

Hodgson, B. B., & Kizior R. J. (2010). *Saunders nursing drug handbook 2010*. St. Louis, MO: Saunders Elsevier.

Infection Control Today. (2005). Aseptic technique and the sterile field. Retrieved on November 2, 2010, from www.infectioncontroltoday.com/articles/2005/04/aseptic-technique-*amp-the-sterile-field.aspx*

Infection, asepsis, and sterile techniques. Retrieved on November 2, 2010, from www.medtrng.com/blackboard/infection_asepsis.htm

Introduction to aseptic technique. Retrieved on November 7, 2010, from www.engenderhealth.org/ip/aseptic/index.html

Jett, J. (2009). *Patient controlled analgesia (PCA) pump*. Shreveport, LA: Louisiana State University Health Sciences Center.

Joint Commission International. (2010). *Joint Commission International accreditation standards for hospitals: Standards lists version* (4th ed.). Oak Brook, IL: Author.

Joint Commission on Accreditation of Healthcare Organizations. (2004). *Health care at the crossroads: Strategies for narrowing the organ donation gap and protection patients*. Oakbrook, IL: Author.

Kerner, D. (2007). Arterial pressure monitoring. Retrieved on November 2, 2010, from www.northshorelij.com/cs/Satellite?c=Document_C&cid=1228246196369&pagename=NSLIJ%2FDocument_C%2FNSLIJ%2FSubTemplate%2Fdocumentwrapper

Kirchman, M. (2010). *Intracranial pressure monitoring and drainage of cerebrospinal fluid via ventricular catheter*. Retrieved on December 5, 2010, from www.home.smh.com/sections/services-procedures/medlib/nursing/NursPandP/crc10_intracranial_041910.pdf

Krishna, M., & Zacharowski, K. (2009). Principles of intra-aortic balloon pump counterpulsation. Retrieved December 6, 2010, from http:/www.medscape.com/viewarticle/587246_print

Lee, T. (2009). *IV therapy*. Mobile, AL: Springhill Medical Center.

Martin, B. (2010). *AACN practice alert: Oral care for patients at risk for ventilator-associated pneumonia* (Rev. ed.). Aliso Viejo, CA: American Association of Critical-Care Nurses.

McDermott, W. (2009). General nursing cares for a patient on CRRT. Retrieved on December 1, 2010, from http://intensivecare.hsnet.

nsw.gov.au/five/doc/hornsby/General%20nursing%20cares%20
fro%20CRRT.Oct06.pdf

Mckenzie, N. Power of attorney. In *Encyclopedia of surgery*. Retrieved on July 26, 2010, from www.surgeryencyclopedia. com/Pa-St/Power-of-Attorney.html

MedicineNet. Retrieved on July 26, 2010, from www.medterms. com/script/main/art.asp?articlekey=4181

Merriam-Webster Online Dictionary. Retrieved on July 20, 2010, from www.merriam-webster.com/dictionary/malpractice

Mobile Infirmary Medical Center. (n.d.). *Dialysis*. Mobile, AL: Author.

Mobile Infirmary Medical Center. (n.d.). *Removal of pulmonary artery catheter (Swan Ganz)*. Mobile, AL: Author.

Mobile Infirmary Medical Center. (n.d.). *Ventilators*. Mobile, AL: Author.

Mullens, A. (2008, November). HNE area intensive care, practice guideline, IABP intra-aortic balloon pump: Medical issues for ICU. Retrieved on December 10, 2010, from http://www.philip-pelefevre.com/JHH-ICU-guidelines/equipment/IABP.pdf

Nador, R., & Lien, D. (2010). Heart—Lung transplantation. In: S. Hunt (Ed.), *UpToDate*. Waltham, MA: UpToDate.

National Guideline Clearinghouse. (2008). Standard precautions in hospitals. In *Prevention and control of healthcare-associated infectious diseases in Massachusetts*. Retrieved on November 10, 2010, from www.guidelines.gov/content.aspx?id=12917&search= isolation+precautions

Nettina, S. M. (2010). *Lippincott manual of nursing practice* (9th ed.). Ambler, PA: Wolters Kluwer Health, Lippincott Williams & Wilkins.

Neuro-ICU Monitoring Techniques. Retrieved on December 10, 2010, from www.columbianeuroicu.org/monitoring-techniques.html

North Shore University Hospital, End Stage Renal Disease Program. (n.d.). *Continuous renal replacement therapy using prisma*. Manhasset, NY: Author.

Northwestern Memorial Hospital. (2007). *Total parenteral nutrition: Discharge instructions*. Chicago, IL: Author.

Nurse Bob's MICU/CCU Survival Guide: Critical Care Concepts, General Nursing Requirements for the Intensive Care Patient. Retrieved October 18, 2010, from www.micunursing.com/gen-eralnursingprotocolforcriticalcare.htm

Olshansky, B. (2010). Temporary cardiac pacing. In D. S. Basow (Ed.), *UpToDate*. Waltham, MA.

Parkland Health & Hospital System Nursing Service. (2009). *Urinary catheterization of the adult*. Retrieved October 13, 2010, from www.parklandhospital.com/other_services/pdf/35_03.pdf

Patient Self Determination Act of 1990. 42 U.S. Code 1395 cc (a), Subpart E-Miscellaneous. Washington, DC: Author.

Paunovic, B., & Sharma, S. (2010). Pulmonary artery catheterization. Retrieved on November 17, 2010, from www.emedicine.medscape.com/article/1824547-print

Pear, S. (2007). Oral care is critical care: The role of oral care in the prevention of hospital-acquired pneumonia. *Infection Control Today*. Retrieved on September 26, 2010, from www.infection-controltoday.com

Pennsylvania Medical Society & The Hospital & Healthsystem Association of Pennsylvania. (2007). *Decide for yourself: A guide to advance health care directives*. Harrisburg, PA: Author.

Powner, D. J., Darby, J. M., & Kellum, J. A. (2004). Proposed treatment guidelines for donor care. *Progress in Transplantation, 14*(1), 16–26. Retrieved on July 31, 2010, from www.natcol.org/prof_development/files/ProposedTreatmentGuidelines.pdf

Quan, K. (2010). *How to perform a head to toe assessment*. Retrieved on August 22, 2010, from www.thenursingsite.com/Articles/Head%20to%20toe%20assessment.html

Recommended practices for maintaining a sterile field. (2006). *AORN Journal*. Retrieved on November 2, 2010, from www.findarticles.com/p/articles/mi_m0FSL/is_2_83/ai_n26857827/?tag=content;col1

Rinehart, W., Hurd, C., & Sloan, D. (2010). *NCLEX-RN exam prep: Care of the client with respiratory disorders*. Indianapolis, IN: Pearson. Retrieved on November 22, 2010, from www.informit.com/articles/printerfriendly.aspx?p=1636985

Ross, M. (2000). *Declogging feeding tubes with pancreatic enzymes*. Retrieved on October 24, 2010, from www.healthcare.uiowa.edu/pharmacy/rxupdate/2000/11RXU.html

Rowlett, R. (2000). *Glasgow Coma Scale*. Retrieved on December 22, 2010, from www.unc.edu/~rowlett/units/scales.glasgow.htm

Rudow, D. L., & Goldstein, M. J. (2008). Critical care management of the liver transplant recipient. *Critical Care Nursing Quarterly*,

232–243. Retrieved on January 7, 2011 from http://www.nurs-ingcenter.com/library/static.asp?pageid=853193

Rushing, J. (2010). Caring for a patient's vascular access for hemo-dialysis. *Nursing, 40*(10), 53.

Saint Thomas Hospital. (2000). *Terminal weaning from ventilator.* Protocol No. V-09. Nashville, TN: Author.

San Diego Patient Safety Taskforce. (2008). *Patient controlled anal-gesia (PCA) guidelines of care: For the opioid naive patient.* San Diego, CA: Author.

Seckel, M. *Implementing evidence-based practice guidelines to mini-mize ventilator-associated pneumonia.* Retrieved on September 21, 2010, from www.aacn.org/WD/CETests/Media/AN0107CE.pdf

Siegel, J. D., Rhinehart, E., Jackson, M., Chiarello, L., & the Healthcare Infection Control Practices Advisory Committee. (2007). *2007 Guidelines for isolation precautions: Preventing trans-mission of infectious agents in healthcare settings.* From www.cdc. gov/hipac/2007IP/isolationprecautions.html

SIMS Portex. (1998). *Tracheostomy Care Handbook: A Guide for the Health Care Provider.* Keene, NH: Author. Retrieved on September 5, 2010, from www.tracheostomy.com/resources/pdf/TrachHandbk.pdf

Springhill Medical Center, Cardiac Catheterization Laboratory. (2010). *Consent titles for cath lab patients.* Mobile, AL: Author.

Springhill Medical Center. (2005). *IV's: Use of local anesthetic.* Mobile, AL: Author.

Springhill Medical Center. (2008). *Approved list for pediatric patients ages 1 month–17 years.* Mobile, AL: Author.

Springhill Medical Center. (2010). *Informed consent.* Mobile, AL: Author.

St. Andre, A., & DelRossi, A. (2005). Hemodynamic management of patients in the first 24 hours after cardiac surgery. *Critical Care Medicine, 33*(90), 2082–2094.

St. Luke's Episcopal Hospital, Texas Heart Institute. (n.d.). ABIOMED BVS 5000. Retrieved on December 6, 2010, from http://www.texasheartinstitute.org/Research/Devices/abiomed.cfm

St. Luke's Episcopal Hospital, Texas Heart Institute. (n.d.). Impella recover LD/LP 5.0 Retrieved on December 6, 2010, from http:/texasheartinstitute.org/Research/Devices/impella.cfm?&RenderForPrint=1

St. Luke's Episcopal Hospital, Texas Heart Institute. (n.d.). Intra-aortic balloon pump. Retrieved on December 6, 2010, from http://www.texasheartinstitute.org/Research/Devices/iabp.cfm

St. Luke's Episcopal Hospital, Texas Heart Institute. (n.d.). Thoratec HeartMate II LVAS. Retrieved on December 6, 2010, from http://www.texasheartinstitute.org/Research/Devices?thoratec_hertmateii.cfm

St. Luke's Episcopal Hospital, Texas Heart Institute. Thoratec HeartMate XVE LVAS. Retrieved December 6, 2010, from www.texasheartinstitute.org/Research/Devices/thoratec.cfm

Staging pressure ulcers. (2010). Retrieved on October 16, 2010, from www.medicaledu.com/staging.htm

Stillwell, S. B. (2006). *Mosby's critical care nursing reference* (4th ed.). St. Louis, MO: Mosby Elsevier.

Swan-Ganz catheterization: Interpretation of tracings. Retrieved on November 17, 2010, from www.personal.health.usf.edu/msiddiqu/Swan.html

U.S. Department of Veterans Affairs, Veterans Health Administration. (2009). *Organ, tissue, and eye donation process. VHA Handbook,* 1101.03. Washington, DC: Author.

Ukleja, A., Freeman, K., Gilbert, K., Kochevar, M., Kraft, M. D., Russell, M. K., et al. (2010). *Standards for nutrition support: Adult hospitalized patients.* Retrieved on October 24, 2010, from www.nutritioncare.org/wcontent.aspx?id=5410

United Network for Organ Sharing. Common myths of organ donation. (2004). Retrieved on July 26, 2010, from www.unos.org/inTheNews/factsheets.asp

United Network for Organ Sharing. Waiting List Candidates. (2010). Retrieved on July 16, 2010, from www.unos.org/

University of Connecticut Health Center, John Dempsey Hospital, Department of Nursing. (2009). Protocol for: Continuous Renal Replacement Therapy (CRRT): Care of the patient. Retrieved on December 1, 2010, from http://nursing.uchc.edu/unit_manuals/intensive_care/docs/CRRTprotocol%20-%20ICU.hemo-Modified.pdf

University of Miami, Leonard M. Miller School of Medicine, Department of Surgery, Life Alliance Organ Recovery Agency. *Benefits of organ and tissue donation.* Retrieved on July 26, 2010, from www.surgery.med.miami.edu/x282.xml

University of Miami, Leonard M. Miller School of Medicine, Department of Surgery, Life Alliance Organ Recovery Agency. *Myth versus fact*. Retrieved on July 26, 2010, from www.surgery. med.miami.edu/x286.xml

University of Miami, Leonard M. Miller School of Medicine, Department of Surgery, Life Alliance Organ Recovery Agency. *The organ donation process*. Retrieved on July 26, 2010, from www.surgery.med.miami.edu/x297.xml

Wingate, S., & Wiegand, D. L. (2008). End-of-life care in the critical care unit for patients with heart failure. *Critical Care Nurse, 28*(2), 84–88, 90–95.

Wyckoff, M., Houghton, D., & LePage, C. (Eds.). (2009). *Critical care concepts, role, and practice for the acute care nurse practitioner*. New York: Springer Publishing.

Index

Visit www.springerpub.com to order.